Rogalla P., Mutze S., Hamm B.
Body CT
State-of-the-Art

MALLINCKRODT
MEDICAL

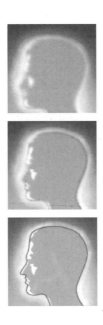

OPTIMIZING
THE PRACTICE OF
MEDICINE

Rogalla P., Mutze S., Hamm B.

Body CT

State-of-the-Art

Protocols for:
Long-spiral CT
Short-spiral CT
Incremental CT

W. Zuckschwerdt Verlag
München · Bern · Wien · New York

Corresponding address:

Patrik Rogalla, M. D.

Department of Radiology
Charité Hospital
Humboldt-Universität zu Berlin
Schumannstrasse 20/21
10098 Berlin, Germany

Special thanks to Bettina Herwig and Noga Meiri for their assistance with translating this book.

Distributors

Germany:	Switzerland:	Austria:	USA:
Brockhaus Kommission	Hans Huber Verlag	Maudrich Verlag	Scholium International Inc.
Verlagsauslieferung	Längassstrasse 76	Spitalgasse 21a	14 Vanderventer Ave
Kreidlerstrasse 9	CH-3000 Bern	A-1097 Wien	Port Washington
D-70806 Kornwestheim			11050 NewYork

Die Deutsche Bibliothek – CIP-Einheitsaufnahme

Rogalla, Patrik: Body CT: state-of-the-art ; protocols for long-spiral CT, short-spiral CT, incremental CT / Rogalla, P. ; Mutze, S. ; Hamm, B. – München ; Bern ; Wien ; New York : Zuckschwerdt, 1996
ISBN 3-88603-565-4
NE: Mutze, Sven ; Hamm, Bernd

© 1996 by W. Zuckschwerdt Verlag GmbH, Industriestrasse 17, D-82110 Germering / München.
Printed in Germany by Presse-Druck Augsburg.

ISBN 3-88603-565-4

Contents

Preface

Computed tomography has undergone dramatic developments since its first introduction into clinical practice. Despite competition with magnetic resonance imaging, computed tomography still is the modality of choice for many diagnostic problems in the area of the trunk. The advent of new scanning techniques such as spiral or helical CT has even reversed the trend towards MRI, with a return to computed tomography in some areas.

Spiral CT not only improves the diagnostic yield, but also opens up new areas of examination. The speed of spiral scanning makes it necessary to carefully plan an examination beforehand, since there are considerable differences among the various indications. Such individual planning brings a totally new quality to computed tomography.

The administration of intravenous contrast material has become part of the standard protocol for most examinations by computed tomography. The increasing speed of the scanners makes it possible to excellently opacify all vessels in the examination area with a single bolus injection of contrast material. The rapidity, furthermore, improves tumor and lesion detection and has led to an optimization of the protocols for contrast agent administration.

The purpose of this book is to serve physicians working in computed tomography as a practical guide for establishing their own examination protocols. The protocols compiled here for different indications and for the three most important scanner types (scanners with a long spiral, scanners with a short spiral, and incremental scanners) have been developed and tested in a routine clinical setting. Our aim was to present the protocols in a clearly arranged manner for quick reference, which is further facilitated by a short summary of each protocol for orientation.

The authors would be glad if this book turns out to be a helpful reference manual for clinicians and practitioners. Any constructive criticism or suggestions for optimizing the CT protocols presented are welcome.

Patrik Rogalla, M. D.
Sven Mutze, M. D.
Bernd Hamm, M. D.

General remarks

All protocols presented have been developed and tested in clinical routine on the following scanners:

General Electric 9800, HiSpeed Advantage
Imatron C100 XL
Philips SR 4000, SR 7000
Picker PQ 2000
Siemens Somatom DR2, DRG/DRH, Plus, Plus S

Unfortunately, there is at present no uniform terminology for the physical parameters and scanning techniques in computed tomography. All manufacturers use their own terms and designations. The authors therefore decided to use the terminology most current in clinical usage. The most important synonyms are given in the following list:

Scout view: topogram, scanogram, pilot scan
Spiral CT: helical CT, volume scan
Incremental CT: axial mode, conventional CT, normal scan
Table feed: (table) index, increment
Slice thickness: collimation, (section) thickness

There are no clear criteria that distinguish short- from long-spiral CT. The term "short-spiral CT" is used in this book for scanners with a maximum of 32 revolutions and "long-spiral CT" for all scanners with a spiral length of more than 32 revolutions.

Determination of beam collimation

All spiral CT scanners presently available permit a beam collimation of 10 mm. For general applicability, the protocols for long-spiral CT recommend to use 10 mm beam collimation, unless explicitly stated otherwise. Generally, however, a narrower beam collimation combined with a higher pitch appears to be preferable since the slice profile is slightly wider in the spiral mode compared to the incremental mode. The following combinations of settings (beam collimation/table increment/reconstruction interval) are nearly equivalent:

10/10/8 = 8/10/8   (pitch 1.25:1)
         = 7/10/7   (pitch 1.4:1)

10/10/4 = 8/10/4   (pitch 1.25:1)
         = 7/10/3.5 (pitch 1.4:1)

5/5/5   = 4/4/4   (pitch 1:1)
         = 4/5/4   (pitch 1.25:1)

5/5/3   = 4/4/3   (pitch 1:1)
         = 4/5/3   (pitch 1.25:1)

Scanning direction

Many protocols for long- and short-spiral CT recommend scanning from bottom to top. This scanning direction avoids beam-hardening artifacts in the area of the upper thoracic aperture caused by the influx of fresh, highly concentrated contrast material. Bottom to top scanning of the liver ensures better opacification of the liver veins, which are examined at the end of the spiral. For details, refer to the remarks under each protocol.

Photography

The window and level (W/L) settings for bone, lung, and soft-tissue vary depending on the scanner, monitor, printer, and type of film. We encourage settings of 400/50 for soft-tissue, 1300/-500 for lung, and 1700/300 for bone.

Intravenous contrast material

All intravenous contrast agents presently approved for computed tomography contain iodine bound in a complex organic molecule. Non-ionic contrast agents are tolerated well, and severe allergic reactions are extremely rare. Data in the literature range from an incidence of 1:10,000 to 1:100,000.

Rapid bolus injection of the formerly used ionic contrast agents led to nausea in some cases, with the patient having to vomit exactly at the optimal time for starting the examination. Since this side-effect is very rare when non-ionic contrast material is used, the former requirement to perform the examination on an empty stomach can now be handled less strictly. Nevertheless, a stomach filled with food is disadvantageous for oral opacification and may considerably impair assessment of the gastric wall.

Briefly informing the patient that a general sensation of warmth throughout the body along with a metallic taste is to be expected shortly after the start of the injection will reassure the patient and prevent misinterpretation. Typically, an antecubital flexible cannula with a diameter of 0.8 mm (22 gauge) will be sufficient in patients who tolerated the contrast agent well in a preceding test. In patients who receive intravenous contrast material for the first time, we recommend inserting a 1 mm cannula (20 gauge) as a precautionary measure in case of an allergic shock reaction that requires fluid substitution.

Power injection is generally preferable to manual injection, especially because higher injection rates are difficult to achieve homogeneously by hand and are rarely reproducible. Most commercially available injectors allow definition of various programs, which can be named after the CT protocols for which they are to be used. A critical phase in automatic contrast material administration occurs at the start of the injection: the more or less sudden onset of the injection may lead to the rupture of thin and fragile veins. Monitoring of the cannula by a physician during this phase is therefore of utmost importance, since patients who receive non-ionic contrast material very rarely report burning or a sensation of pain at the injection site.

The indicated scan delay times after starting the injection of contrast material are mean values which typically result in optimal opacification in patients with normal cardiac function. However, since there are considerable variations in circulation times, the scan delay times may have to be even twice as long in patients with severe heart failure. Individual measurements of circulation times for computed tomography appear to be imperative; currently, only General Electric offers a software solution as an additional package for spiral CT scanners.

Premedication

Patients who are known to be highly susceptible to allergic reactions or have previously had adverse reactions to contrast material require premedication prior to injection of an intravenous contrast agent. Numerous recommendations have been made; the following drugs and dosages are only one variant among them:

− Prednisone 40 mg orally 12 and 2 hours prior to study
− H1-receptor blocker: Benadryl® 50 mg orally one hour prior to study

Alternatives to iodine-containing contrast agents

If there are strict contraindications to the administration of iodine-containing contrast material, for instance in patients scheduled for radio-iodine treatment, gadolinium-DTPA (Gd-DTPA) can be used as an alternative. Since Gd-DTPA has only one gadolinium atom per molecule – as opposed to contrast agents with 3 iodine atoms per molecule – its radiodensity is only about 35% of that of iodine-containing contrast agents. Currently, administration of more than 60 ml of Gd-DTPA appears to be clinically unacceptable. Two protocols using Gd-DTPA for neck and chest studies are suggested at the end of the book.

Oral and rectal contrast material

Two basic types of contrast agents are available for oral and rectal application: iodine-containing water solutions and barium sulfate suspensions. Both types are used equally in clinical routine, and no severe side-effects have been reported with proper dosage. Nevertheless, there are slight pharmacological and physical differences between these two agents, which speak in favor of iodine solutions:

1. Iodine-containing solutions have a mild positive effect on bowel peristalsis, resulting in a more rapid passage of the contrast material to distal ileum loops, occurring within 30–60 minutes after oral administration. Disadvantage: There are rare cases of mild diarrhea.

2. Iodine-containing solutions show a more homogeneous distribution in the bowel and, unlike barium sulfate, do not tend to undergo flocculation. Large barium lumps may become so radiodense that they produce artifacts and thus obscure wall pathology.

3. In some patients, barium sulfate leads to circular mural thickening, primarily in distal segments of the small bowel, which may be misdiagnosed as enteritis. A possible underlying mechanism of this phenomenon is the hydrophilic nature of barium sulfate suspensions, which leads to edematous swelling of the mucosa.

4. Patients with suspected perforation who are scheduled for bowel surgery should only receive iodine-containing contrast material.

Administration of one liter of contrast material over a period of one hour prior to the examination has been shown to be most effective. Some radiologists administer 20 mg of metoclopramide (MCP®, 2 tablets) with the first cup of contrast material to accelerate its passage. This typically shortens the contrast administration period to half an hour. Side-effects of MCP – diarrhea and muscle tremor – are unlikely to occur after administration of a single dose.

The application of rectal contrast material – the same substances as those for oral use are available – is a stressful and time-consuming procedure for both patients and physicians. It may be painful to introduce the rectal probe in patients with hemorrhoids, and feelings of shame have to be overcome in some patients. Nevertheless, rectal contrast material should be administered for all examinations of the pelvis, unless there are contraindications such as neutropenia, anal carcinoma, or deep-seated rectal carcinoma. In these cases, or if such a tumor is suspected, a preceding digital examination is necessary to avoid iatrogenic perforation by too forceful and uncontrolled insertion of the rigid probe.

We recommend to use ready-made enema bags containing about 500 – 1000 ml of iodine- or barium-containing contrast material. It is normally easier for the patients to retain the fluid in the bowel if the probe is left in the rectum during the examination. It can then also be used to remove the fluid after scanning.

Respiration during the examination

For the sake of uniformity, all examinations are performed during inspiration. Although the level of inspiration is defined more precisely during expiration and is easier to reproduce by the patients, most patients can hold their breath much longer in inspiration. A long breath-hold without respiratory movements is, in particular, advantageous for spiral CT examinations. However, studies have shown that the spiral technique is less susceptible to artifacts than conventional CT. Even smooth, continuous breathing during scanning has only a negligible effect on image quality. Examinations of the upper thoracic aperture and of the pelvis require only minimal cooperation from the patient.

Radiation exposure

A considerable proportion of the radiation exposure in medicine is caused by computed tomography, about 30% according to recent data. Besides strictly limiting the indication for computed tomography, the following measures can help to reduce radiation exposure:

1. Reduction of the energy (mA) to a minimal level. This is achieved at the expense of increased image noise.

2. Elevation of the pitch factor (ratio of table feed to slice thickness). A 50% increase of the table feed at a constant nominal slice thickness will reduce the radiation dose by 33%. At the same time, however, this measure increases the effective section thickness up to 50%.

3. Precise determination of the area to be examined. The use of pre-programmed spirals often yields unnecessary scans, since a spiral, once started, is not intended to be stopped before completion.

4. Storage of raw data sets. In all unclear cases, these data can be used to calculate images with different kernels or magnifications, or, for spiral CT, images with a different reconstruction interval even days after the examination. However, this requires a considerable storage capacity.

Long-spiral CT

Abdomen and pelvis

Region	above diaphragm to pubic symphysis
Scout view	500 mm, 120 kV, 50–100 mA, pa
Contrast media	i.v.: 120 ml non-ionic CM, iodine content: 300–320 mg/ml oral: 1000 ml over 60 min rectal: 500 ml immediately before scanning
Injection rate	2.5 ml/sec
Scan delay time	50 sec after start of bolus
CT technique	120 kV, 175–300 mA, 512 matrix, inspiration 1st spiral: 10 mm slice thickness / 10 mm table feed (pitch 1:1) bottom to top, tip of liver to above diaphragm 2nd spiral: 10 mm slice thickness / 10 mm table feed (pitch 1:1) bottom to top, symphysis to tip of liver
Reconstruction	8 mm interval for both spirals, soft-tissue algorithm
Photography	12 on 1, patient information, scout view without and with cut lines, soft-tissue window from top to bottom, basal lung segments at lung window (with edge enhancement if necessary)
Remarks	1. Overlap first section of the 1st spiral with last section of the 2nd spiral. 2. Have the patient drink a cup of water immediately before scanning for better filling of the stomach. 3. Instruct the patient to breathe deeply before scanning. 4. If post-processing in 2D (multiplanar)/3D is required, the reconstruction interval should be 3 mm (approx. 30% of the nominal slice thickness), use identical FOV and matrix for both spirals. 5. The pitch can be increased up to 2:1. 6. In case of a pathologic finding in the kidneys, ureters, or bladder, delayed scanning with 150–200 mA after 5 min may be necessary. 7. Rectal CM administration should be performed for all gynecological examinations and suspected pathology in the colon/rectum. As an alternative to a contrast enema, a pre-packaged implementation device (approx. 150 ml) can be used. 8. Co-administration of 20 mg metoclopramide (MCP) with the first cup of contrast material accelerates the CM passage. 9. For oral and rectal CM administration, see "General remarks", page IX.

Brief protocol

CM oral, rectal
i.v.
120 ml
2.5 ml/sec
50 sec
10/10/8
bottom to top

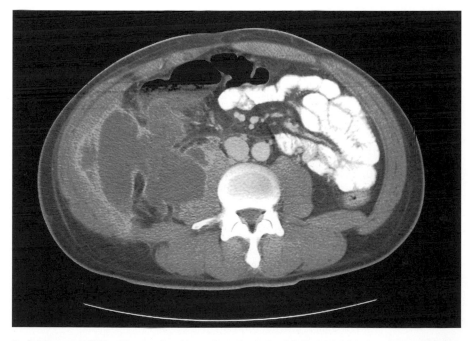

Perforating appendicitis with extensive abscess formation in the right flank involving the psoas muscle. Pronounced rim enhancement of the abscess formation and homogeneous opacification of the inferior vena cava and abdominal aorta.

Chest and upper abdomen

Region	above clavicles to lower kidney pole
Scout view	500 mm, 120 kV, 50–100 mA, pa
Contrast media	i.v.: 120 ml non-ionic CM, iodine content: 300–320 mg/ml oral: 1000 ml over 60 min
Injection rate	2.5 ml/sec
Scan delay time	50 sec after start of bolus
CT technique	120 kV, 75–300 mA, 512 matrix, inspiration 1st spiral: 10 mm slice thickness / 10 mm table feed (pitch 1:1) bottom to top, tip of liver to above diaphragm 2nd spiral: 10 mm slice thickness / 10 mm table feed (pitch 1:1) bottom to top, diaphragm to above clavicles
Reconstruction	8 mm interval, 1st spiral with soft-tissue algorithm, 2nd spiral in lung/bone algorithm
Photography	12 on 1, patient information, scout view without and with cut lines, soft-tissue window from top to bottom, lung window (with edge enhancement if necessary)
Remarks	1. Overlap last section of the 1st spiral with first section of the 2nd spiral. 2. Have the patient drink a cup of water immediately before scanning for better filling of the stomach. 3. Instruct the patient to breathe deeply before scanning. 4. Caudo-cranial sectioning is associated with markedly fewer beam-hardening artifacts at the upper thoracic aperture caused by the influx of fresh, highly concentrated contrast material. 5. If post-processing in 2D (multiplanar)/3D is required, the reconstruction interval should be 3 mm (approx. 30% of the nominal slice thickness), use identical FOV and matrix for both spirals. 6. The pitch can be increased up to 2:1. 7. A suitable contrast agent for the esophagus is Esopho-Cat® (2 tablespoons immediately before scanning). 8. In case of a pathologic finding in the renal pelvis/ureter, delayed scanning after 5 min may be necessary. 9. For oral CM administration, see "General remarks", page IX.

Brief protocol

CM oral, i.v.
120 ml
2.5 ml/sec
50 sec
10/10/8
bottom to top

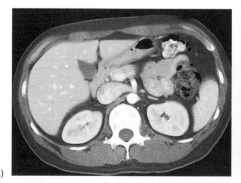

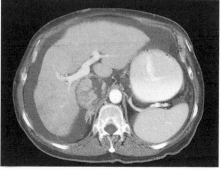

a)

b)

(a) Artifact: heterogeneous opacification of the inferior vena cava caused by mixing of non-opacified blood from the lower region of the body with opacified renal vein blood. (b) No artifact: heterogeneous opacification of the inferior vena cava due to intracaval leiomyosarcoma with extensive thrombus formation.

Neck and chest

Region	below base of skull to below both sinuses of dlaphragm include adrenals in bronchogenic carcinoma
Scout view	chest: 400 mm, 120 kV, 50–100 mA, pa neck: 250 mm, 120 kV, 50–100 mA, lateral
Contrast media	i.v.: 80 ml (chest) + 40 ml (neck) non-ionic CM, iodine content: 300–320 mg/ml
Injection rate	2 ml/sec for chest and neck bolus
Scan delay time	30 sec after start of bolus for chest, 20 sec after start of neck bolus
CT technique	120 kV, 75–200 mA, inspiration 1st spiral: 10 mm slice thickness / 10 mm table feed (pitch 1:1) bottom to top, sinus to above clavicles reposition patient with arms parallel to trunk, inclince gantry parallel to inter-vertebral disc C4–C5, start neck bolus 2nd spiral: 5 mm slice thickness / 5 mm table feed (pitch 1:1) bottom to top, above clavicles to base of skull
Reconstruction	4 mm interval for 1st spiral, lung/bone algorithm 5 mm interval for 2nd spiral, soft-tissue algorithm
Photography	12 on 1, patient information, scout view without and with cut lines, all ima-ges of the 2nd spiral and alternate images of the 1st spiral at soft-tissue win-dow from top to bottom, lung window from top to bottom (with edge enhance-ment if necessary)
Remarks	1. Overlap last section of the 1st spiral with first section of the 2nd spiral. 2. Most patients can hold their breath for up to 25 sec. Respiratory excursions in the upper part of the chest have little effect on image quality. Instruct the patient to avoid sudden (respiratory) movements. 3. Caudo-cranial sectioning is associated with markedly fewer beam-harden-ing artifacts at the upper thoracic aperture caused by the influx of fresh, high-ly concentrated contrast material. 4. For indications without search for intrapulmonary nodules smaller than 3 mm, the reconstruction interval can be increased to 8 mm. 5. A suitable contrast agent for the esophagus is Esopho-Cat® (2 tablespoons immediately before scanning). 6. If post-processing in 2D (multiplanar)/3D is required, the reconstruction inter-val should be 3 mm (approx. 30% of the nominal slice thickness).

7. The pitch can be increased up to 2:1.
8. Edge enhancement (implemented in most scanners as a post-processing function) facilitates the detection of very small lung lesions.
9. Follow-up of intrapulmonary nodules during therapy may be done without intravenous administration of contrast material.
10. The tube current should be reduced to 50 mA in slender patients.

Brief protocol
CM i.v.
80/40 ml
2 ml/sec
30/20 sec
10/10/4, 5/5/5
bottom to top

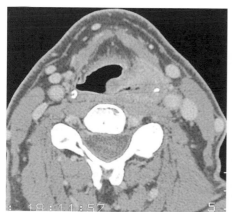 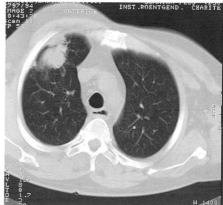

Hypopharyngeal carcinoma on the left. Intravenous injection of contrast material results in heterogeneous enhancement of the tumor and facilitates assessment of the lymph nodes. Metastasis of the hypopharyngeal carcinoma in the right upper lobe of the lung.

Chest, abdomen, and pelvis

Region	above clavicles to pubic symphysis
Scout view	600 mm, 120 kV, 50–100 mA, pa
Contrast media	i.v.: 120 ml (abdomen and pelvis) + 40 ml (chest) non-ionic CM, iodine content: 300–320 mg/ml oral: 1000 ml over 60 min rectal: 500 ml immediately before scanning
Injection rate	2.5 ml/sec for abdomen and pelvis, 2 ml/sec for chest bolus
Scan delay time	50 sec after start of bolus, 20 sec after start of chest bolus
CT technique	120 kV, 75–300 mA, 512 matrix, inspiration 1st spiral: 10 mm slice thickness / 10 mm table feed (pitch 1:1) bottom to top, tip of liver to above diaphragm 2nd spiral: 10 mm slice thickness / 10 mm table feed (pitch 1:1) bottom to top, symphysis to tip of liver reconstruct images or store on hard disc, depending on scanner type; start chest bolus 3rd spiral: 10 mm slice thickness / 10 mm table feed (pitch 1:1) bottom to top, sinus to above clavicles
Reconstruction	8 mm interval for all spirals, soft-tissue algorithm for 1st and 2nd spiral, lung/bone algorithm for 3rd spiral
Photography	12 on 1, patient information, scout view without and with cut lines, soft-tissue window from top to bottom, lung window (with edge enhancement if necessary)
Remarks	1. Overlap one section between adjacent spirals. 2. Have the patient drink a cup of water immediately before scanning for better filling of the stomach. 3. Instruct the patient to breathe deeply before scanning. 4. If post-processing in 2D (multiplanar)/3D is required, the reconstruction interval should be 3 mm (approx. 30% of the nominal slice thickness), use identical FOV and matrix for all spirals. 5. The pitch can be increased up to 2:1. 6. In case of a pathologic finding in the kidneys, ureters, or bladder, delayed scanning with 150–200 mA after 5 min may be necessary. 7. Rectal CM administration should be performed for all gynecological examinations and suspected pathology in the colon/rectum. As an alternative to

	Brief protocol
	CM oral, rectal
	i.v.
	120/40 ml
	2.5/2 ml/sec
	50/20 sec
	10/10/8
	bottom to top

a contrast enema, a pre-packaged implementation device (approx. 150 ml) can be used.

8. Co-administration of 20 mg metoclopramide (MCP) with the first cup of contrast material accelerates the CM passage.
9. The protocol can be changed for scanners with a spiral length > 60 cm or if the pitch is increased to 1.5:1: 10/10/8 through the liver, 10/10/8 through the chest, followed by 10/10/8 through the pelvis without additional contrast administration. CM administration: 150 ml, 2 ml/sec, 50 sec scan delay.
10. A separate examination of the chest and abdomen/pelvis is recommended for fine assessment.
11. For oral and rectal CM administration, see "General remarks", page IX.

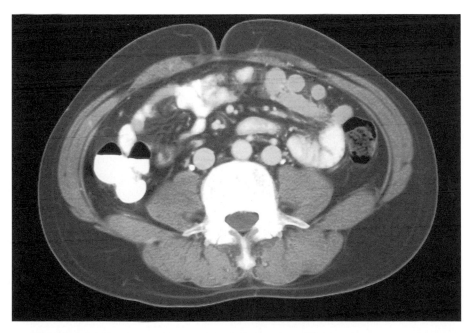

Doubling of the inferior vena cava. Adequate arterial opacification is maintained until the end of the second spiral.

Neck, chest, abdomen, and pelvis

Region	below base of skull to pubic symphysis
Scout view	trunk: 600 mm, 120 kV, 50–100 mA, pa neck: 250 mm, 120 kV, 50–100 mA, lateral
Contrast media	i.v.: 110 ml (abdomen and pelvis) + 40 ml (chest) + 30 ml (neck) non-ionic CM, iodine content: 300–320 mg/ml oral: 1000 ml over 60 min rectal: 500 ml immediately before scanning
Injection rate	2.5 ml/sec for abdomen and pelvis, 2 ml/sec for chest bolus, 1.5 ml/sec for neck bolus
Scan delay time	50 sec after start of 1st bolus, 20 sec after start of chest bolus 15 sec after start of neck bolus
CT technique	120 kV, 75–300 mA, 512 matrix, inspiration 1st spiral: 10 mm slice thickness / 10 mm table feed (pitch 1:1) bottom to top, tip of liver to above diaphragm 2nd spiral: 10 mm slice thickness / 10 mm table feed (pitch 1:1) bottom to top, symphysis to tip of liver reconstruct images or store on hard disc, depending on scanner type; start chest bolus 3rd spiral: 10 mm slice thickness / 10 mm table feed (pitch 1:1) bottom to top, sinus to above clavicles reconstruct images or store on hard disc, depending on scanner type; reposition patient's arms, start neck bolus 4th spiral: 5 mm slice thickness / 5 mm table feed (pitch 1:1) bottom to top, above clavicles to base of skull
Reconstruction	8 mm interval for spirals 1–3, spirals 1 and 2 with soft-tissue algorithm, spiral 3 with lung/bone algorithm 5 mm interval for spiral 4, soft-tissue algorithm
Photography	12 on 1, patient information, scout view without and with cut lines, soft-tissue window from top to bottom, lung window (with edge enhancement if necessary)
Remarks	1. Since the chest and abdomen bolus may obscure neck pathology (tumors), we recommend to examine the neck or chest/neck separately from the abdomen/pelvis (at least 6 hours apart).

2. Overlap one section between adjacent spirals.
3. Have the patient drink a cup of water immediately before scanning for better filling of the stomach.
4. The pitch can be increased up to 2:1.
5. In case of a pathologic finding in the kidneys, ureters, or bladder, delayed scanning with 150–200 mA after 5 min may be necessary.
6. Rectal CM administration should be performed for all gynecological examinations and suspected pathology in the colon/rectum. As an alternative to a contrast enema, a pre-packaged implementation device (approx. 150 ml) can be used.

CM oral, rectal i.v.
110/40/30 ml
2.5/2/1.5 ml/sec
50/20/15 sec
10/10/8, 5/5/5
bottom to top

7. The protocol can be changed for scanners with a spiral length > 60 cm or if the pitch is increased to 1.5:1: 10/10/8 through the liver, 10/10/8 through the chest, followed by 10/10/8 through the pelvis without additional contrast administration. Reposition the arms, give neck bolus, 5/5/5 through the neck. CM administration: 150 ml, 2 ml/sec, 50 sec scan delay, neck bolus: 30 ml, 1.5 ml/sec, 15 sec scan delay.

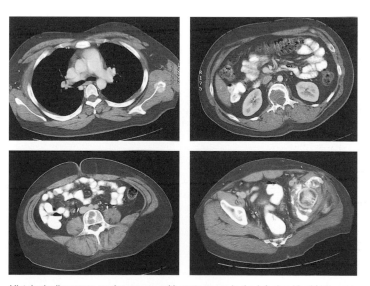

Histologically proven angiosarcoma with metastases in the left shoulder blade, several vertebral bodies, and the left hip joint. A second CM bolus for the 3rd spiral (chest) ensures optimal opacification of the thoracic vessels.

Neck

Region	below base of skull to tip of lung or to above aortic arch if required
Scout view	250 mm, 120 kV, 50–100 mA, lateral
Contrast media	i.v.: 80 ml non-ionic CM, iodine content: 300–320 mg/ml
Injection rate	2 ml/sec
Scan delay time	40 sec after start of bolus
CT technique	120 kV, 75–150 mA, inspiration incline gantry parallel to intervertebral disc C4–C5 spiral: 5 mm slice thickness / 5 mm table feed (pitch 1:1) top to bottom
Reconstruction	5 mm interval, soft-tissue algorithm
Photography	12 on 1, patient information, scout view without and with cut lines, soft-tissue window from top to bottom, scans containing lung segments at lung window from top to bottom (with edge enhancement if necessary)
Remarks	1. For assessment of tumor extension (but not for lymph node staging), the scan delay may be increased to 70 sec and the amount of CM should be 120 ml. 2. Ask the patient not to swallow during the examination. 3. If post-processing in 2D (multiplanar)/3D is required, the reconstruction interval should be 2 mm (approx. 30% of the nominal slice thickness). 4. The pitch can be increased up to 2:1. 5. The tube current should be reduced to 75 mA in patients with a slender neck.

Brief protocol

CM i.v.
80 ml
2 ml/sec
40 sec
5/5/5
top to bottom

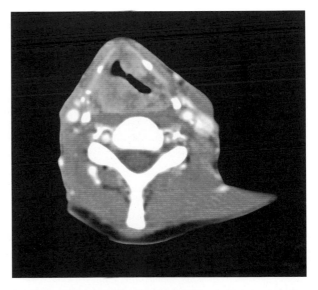

Carcinoma of the larynx. Complete opacification of all arteries and veins makes it possible to assess the lymph nodes.

Chest

Region	above clavicles to below both sinuses of diaphragm include adrenals in bronchogenic carcinoma
Scout view	400 mm, 120 kV, 50–100 mA, pa
Contrast media	i.v.: 80 ml non-ionic CM, iodine content: 300–320 mg/ml
Injection rate	2 ml/sec
Scan delay time	30 sec after start of bolus
CT technique	120 kV, 75–200 mA, inspiration spiral: 10 mm slice thickness / 10 mm table feed (pitch 1:1) bottom to top, sinus to above clavicles
Reconstruction	4 mm interval, lung/bone algorithm
Photography	12 on 1, patient information, scout view without and with cut lines, alternate images at soft-tissue window from top to bottom, lung window from top to bottom (with additional edge enhancement if necessary)
Remarks	1. Most patients can hold their breath for up to 25 sec. Respiratory excursions in the upper part of the chest have little effect on image quality. Instruct the patient to avoid sudden (respiratory) movements. 2. Caudo-cranial sectioning is associated with markedly fewer beam-hardening artifacts at the upper thoracic aperture caused by the influx of fresh, highly concentrated contrast material. 3. The reconstruction interval is 4 mm. To keep the number of images to be interpreted within reasonable limits, only alternate images should be photographed (corresponding to a reconstruction interval of 8 mm). In all unclear cases or if a CT scanner with a cine mode is available, the lung can be "leafed through" at the console. 4. For indications without search for intrapulmonary nodules smaller than 3 mm, the reconstruction interval can be increased to 8 mm. 5. A suitable contrast agent for the esophagus is Esopho-Cat® (2 tablespoons immediately before scanning). 6. If post-processing in 2D (multiplanar)/3D is required, the reconstruction interval should be 3 mm (approx. 30% of the nominal slice thickness). 7. The pitch can be increased up to 2:1. 8. Edge enhancement (implemented in most scanners as a post-processing function) facilitates the detection of very small lung lesions. 9. Follow-up of intrapulmonary nodules during therapy may be done without intravenous administration of contrast material. 10. The tube current should be reduced to 50 mA in slender patients.

Brief protocol

CM i.v.
80 ml
2 ml/sec
30 sec
10/10/4
bottom to top

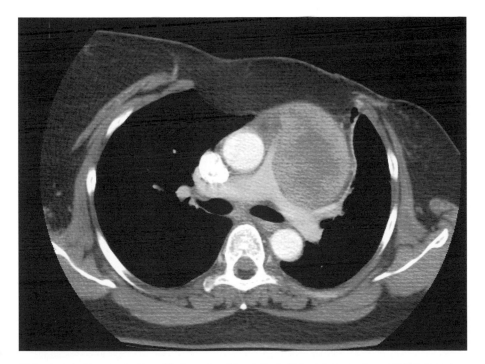

Status post plastic reconstruction of the thoracic wall in a patient with breast cancer, stage pT4. Note the extensive mediastinal tumor recurrence with central necrotic areas and compression of the pulmonary artery trunk. Optimal opacification of all thoracic vessels is necessary for assessment of infiltration.

Chest in HR technique (high-resolution technique)

Region	tip of lung to below both sinuses of diaphragm
Scout view	400 mm, 120 kV, 50–100 mA, pa
Contrast media	–
Injection rate	–
Scan delay time	–
CT technique	140 kV, 75–200 mA, 512 matrix, 1–2 sec scan time, inspiration
	1–2 mm slice thickness / 10 mm table feed top to bottom, allow patient to breathe after 5 scans (≈ 20 sec)
Reconstruction	lung/bone algorithm
Photography	12 on 1, patient information, scout view without and with cut lines, soft-tissue window, lung window
Remarks	1. This protocol can only be used for assessing interstitial pulmonary changes or bronchiectasis. The 8–9 mm interscan gap limits the assessment of mediastinal lymphadenopathy or intrapulmonary nodules. 2. If contrast-enhanced scans are required, use chest protocol in spiral technique. 3. With a scan time of 2 sec per section, more raw data can be acquired than with 1-sec scans, which improves contrast and resolution of details. 4. The tube current should be reduced to 50 mA in slender patients. 5. If subpleurally increased interstitial reticulation (basal/dorsal) is noted, turn patient to prone position and acquire single scans through this area after 5 min (thereby excluding purely orthostatic changes).

Brief protocol

**unenhanced
1–2/10
top to bottom**

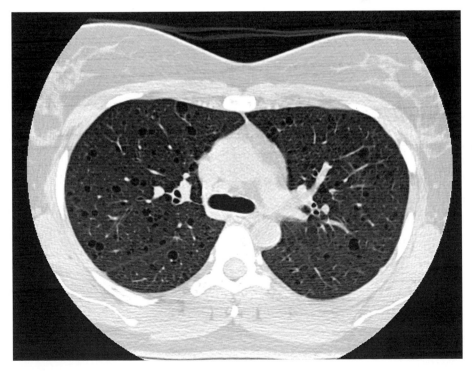

Lymphangiomyomatosis of the lung in a patient with Pringle's disease. Multiple bulla-like structures in all segments.

Upper abdomen

Region	above diaphragm to lower renal pole
Scout view	350 mm, 120 kV, 50–100 mA, pa
Contrast media	i.v.: 120 ml non-ionic CM, iodine content: 300–320 mg/ml oral: 1000 ml over 60 min
Injection rate	2.5 ml/sec
Scan delay time	50 sec after start of bolus
CT technique	120 kV, 175–300 mA, 512 matrix, inspiration spiral: 10 mm slice thickness / 10 mm table feed (pitch 1:1) bottom to top
Reconstruction	8 mm interval, soft-tissue algorithm
Photography	12 on 1, patient information, scout view without and with cut lines, soft-tissue window from top to bottom, basal lung segments at lung window (with edge enhancement if necessary)
Remarks	1. Have the patient drink a cup of water immediately before scanning for better filling of the stomach. 2. Instruct the patient to breathe deeply before scanning. 3. If post-processing in 2D (multiplanar)/3D is required, the reconstruction interval should be 3 mm (approx. 30% of the nominal slice thickness). 4. The pitch can be increased up to 2:1. 5. In case of a pathologic finding in the renal pelvis/ureter, delayed scanning after 5 min may be necessary. 6. For oral CM administration, see "General remarks", page IX.

Brief protocol
CM oral, i.v. 120 ml 2.5 ml/sec 50 sec 10/10/8 bottom to top

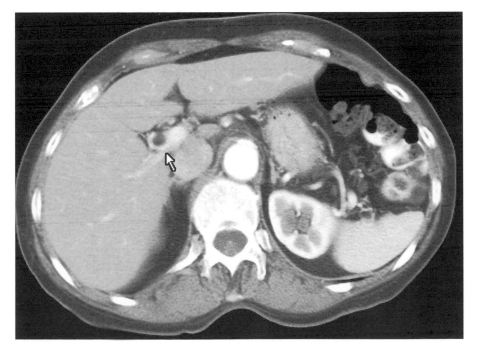

Unclear mass in the porta hepatis seen on ultrasound. Optimal opacification of the portal vein and retrospective reconstruction of the sections through the liver hilus at 3 mm intervals reveals a small fatty protrusion compressing the portal vein.

Pelvis

Region	lower kidney pole to pubic symphysis
Scout view	300 mm, 120 kV, 50–100 mA, pa
Contrast media	i.v.: 120 ml non-ionic CM, iodine content: 300–320 mg/ml oral: 1000 ml over 60 min rectal: 500 ml immediately before scanning
Injection rate	2.5 ml/sec
Scan delay time	70 sec after start of bolus
CT technique	120 kV, 175–300 mA, 512 matrix, inspiration spiral: 10 mm slice thickness / 10 mm table feed (pitch 1:1) top to bottom
Reconstruction	8 mm interval, soft-tissue algorithm
Photography	12 on 1, patient information, scout view without and with cut lines, soft-tissue window from top to bottom
Remarks	1. Beam-hardening artifacts at the level of the hip joints when the bladder is filled with contrast material make it very difficult to assess the pelvic wall in suspected lymphadenopathy. 2. Acquire delayed scans with CM filled bladder only for assessment of bladder pathology. 3. For assessment of suspected pelvic vein thrombosis, the scan delay should be at least 120 sec, and the injection rate should be reduced to 1.5 ml/sec. 4. If post-processing in 2D (multiplanar)/3D is required, the reconstruction interval of the spiral should be 3 mm (approx. 30% of the nominal slice thickness). 5. The pitch can be increased up to 2:1. 6. Minimize energy (< 175 mA) especially in younger patients! 7. Always administer contrast material rectally. As an alternative to a contrast enema, a pre-packaged implementation device (approx. 150 ml) can be used. 8. Co-administration of 20 mg metoclopramide (MCP) with the first cup of contrast material accelerates the CM passage. 9. For oral and rectal CM administration, see "General remarks", page IX.

Brief protocol

CM oral, rectal
i.v.
120 ml
2.5 ml/sec
70 sec
10/10/8
top to bottom

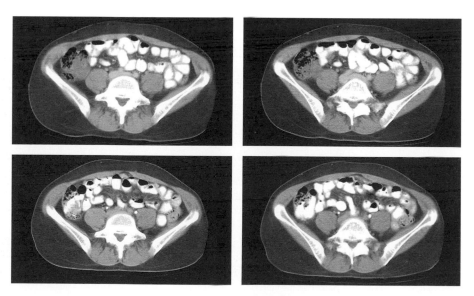

Sonographically suspected cecal tumor; scanning during apparently complete opacification of the bowel demonstrates an unclear cecal mass of 2.5 cm. Delayed scans after 45 minutes following administration of 20 mg MCP reveal the mass to be fecal matter.

Liver (search for lesions of unknown origin)

Region	entire liver
Scout view	350 mm, 120 kV, 50–100 mA, pa
Contrast media	i.v.: 150 ml non-ionic CM, iodine content: 300–320 mg/ml oral: 1000 ml over 60 min
Injection rate	4 ml/sec
Scan delay time	20 sec after start of bolus for arterial phase 60 sec after start of bolus for portal venous phase
CT technique	120 kV, 175–300 mA, 512 matrix, inspiration 1st spiral: 10 mm slice thickness / 10 mm table feed (pitch 1:1) bottom to top 2nd spiral: same location and parameters as 1st spiral
Reconstruction	4 mm interval, soft-tissue algorithm
Photography	12 on 1, patient information, scout view without and with cut lines, only alternate images, both phases at soft-tissue window from top to bottom, basal lung segments of one phase at lung window (with edge enhancement if necessary)
Remarks	1. Two scanning series through the liver during the arterial and during the portal venous phase will detect both hypovascularized and hypervascularized metastases such as metastases from renal cell carcinoma, melanoma, breast cancer, and metastases from endocrine tumors. Small HCCs may also be hypervascularized; they are delineated during the arterial phase and are nearly isodense to liver parenchyma during the portal venous phase. In most cases, this procedure will also demonstrate hemangiomas larger than 1 cm (nodular rim enhancement and fill-in) or cysts (no increase in density). 2. The reconstruction interval is 4 mm. To keep the number of images to be interpreted within reasonable limits, only alternate images should be photographed (corresponding to a reconstruction interval of 8 mm). In all unclear cases or if a CT scanner with a cine mode is available, the liver can be "leafed through" at the console. 3. If post-processsing in 2D (multiplanar)/3D is required, the reconstruction interval should be 3 mm (approx. 30% of the nominal slice thickness). 4. The pitch can be increased up to 2:1. 5. For oral CM administration, see "General remarks", page IX.

Brief protocol
CM oral, i.v.
150 ml
4 ml/sec
20/60 sec
10/10/4
bottom to top

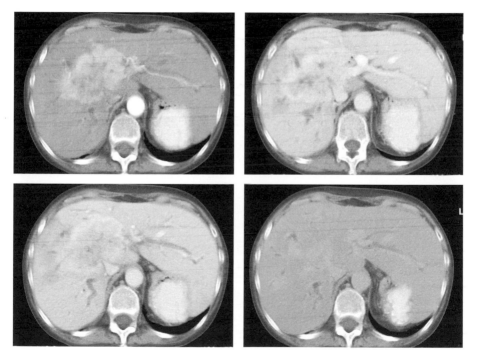

29-year-old female with histologically proven cholangiocellular carcinoma. The notably hypervascularized tumor shows pronounced contrast enhancement in the arterial phase and is already less well delineated during the portal venous phase. The scan after 10 minutes shows the characteristic delayed contrast enhancement, though only to a moderate degree due to the aggressive growth of the tumor.

Liver (search for hypovascularized metastases)

Region	entire liver
Scout view	350 mm, 120 kV, 50–100 mA, pa
Contrast media	i.v.: 120 ml non-ionic CM, iodine content: 300–320 mg/ml oral: 1000 ml over 60 min
Injection rate	2.5 ml/sec
Scan delay time	60 sec after start of bolus (portal venous phase)
CT technique	120 kV, 175–300 mA, 512 matrix, inspiration spiral: 10 mm slice thickness / 10 mm table feed (pitch 1:1) bottom to top
Reconstruction	4 mm interval, soft-tissue algorithm
Photography	12 on 1, patient information, scout view without and with cut lines, alternate images at soft-tissue window from top to bottom, basal lung segments at lung window (with edge enhancement if necessary)
Remarks	1. If hypovascularized metastases are expected, e.g. from adenocarcinoma, scanning during the arterial phase does not yield any additional diagnostic information. 2. The reconstruction interval is 4 mm. To keep the number of images to be interpreted within reasonable limits, only alternate images should be photographed (corresponding to a reconstruction interval of 8 mm). In all unclear cases or if a CT scanner with a cine mode is available, the liver can be "leafed through" at the console. 3. If post-processing in 2D (multiplanar)/3D is required, the reconstruction interval should be 3 mm (approx. 30% of the nominal slice thickness). 4. The pitch can be increased up to 2:1. 5. Obtain delayed scans after 5–10 min in patients with suspected cholangiocarcinoma or gallbladder carcinoma, since these tumors show a characteristic enhancement pattern in the late phase. 6. For oral CM administration, see "General remarks", page IX.

Brief protocol

CM oral, i.v.
120 ml
2.5 ml/sec
60 sec
10/10/4
bottom to top

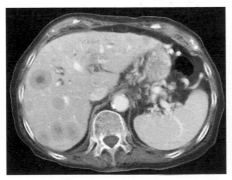 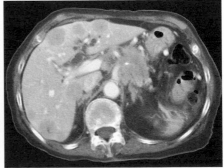

4 cm carcinoma of the pancreatic body with tumorous encasement of the celiac trunk, retroperitoneal lymph-adenopathy, intrahepatic dilatation of the bile ducts, and multiple hypovascularized liver metastases. Scans during the portal venous phase with optimal opacification of the celiac trunk and portal vein.

Liver (lesion characterization)

Region	liver lesion
Scout view	350 mm, 120 kV, 50–100 mA, pa
Unenhanced	120 kV, 75–150 mA, inspiration
	spiral: 10 mm slice thickness / 20 mm table feed (pitch 2:1) top to bottom scanning of the expected liver lesion
Contrast media	i.v.: 120 ml non-ionic CM, iodine content: 300–320 mg/ml no oral contrast material
Injection rate	4 ml/sec
Scan delay time	15 sec after start of bolus (arterial phase)
CT technique	120 kV, 50–210 mA, 512 matrix, inspiration, localize largest extension of lesion, followed by serial dynamic study
	dynamic: 10 mm slice thickness / 0 mm table feed 8 acquisitions every 3 sec, followed by 5 acquisitions every 10 sec, and 1 acquisition each after 2, 3, 4, and 5 min instruct patient to breathe after the initial 8 acquisitions, after the following 3, and then before each of the acquisitions at 1 min intervals
Reconstruction	soft-tissue algorithm
Photography	12 on 1, patient information, scout view without and with cut lines, soft-tissue window
Remarks	1. The dynamic CM enhanced study starting in the early arterial phase yields information for lesion characterization (in particular differentiation of FNH, adenoma, HCC, hemangioma). The patient has to be instructed prior to the examination to attain a similar degree of inspiration with each breath-hold for image acquisition at identical locations. 2. The dynamic study can be evaluated by means of an ROI (region of interest) placed in the lesion and plotting of a time/density curve. 3. The tube current should not exceed 210 mA per scan to minimize radiation exposure. 4. Giant lesions may require delayed scanning after 10 min.

unenhanced
CM i.v.
120 ml
4 ml/sec
15 sec
dynamic series

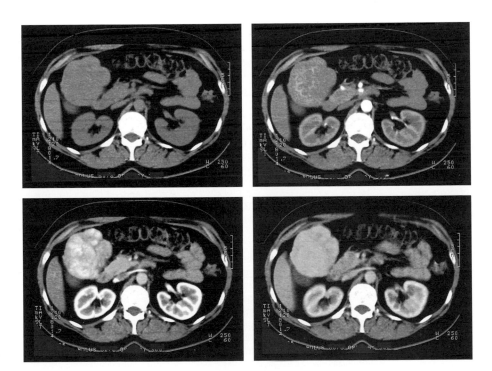

Pedicled hepatocellular carcinoma at the right hepatic lobe. The dynamic study at identical locations shows the heterogeneous, early enhancement initiation of the lesion.

CT during arterial portography (CTAP)

Region	entire liver
Scout view	350 mm, 120 kV, 50–100 mA, pa
Unenhanced	120 kV, 75–150 mA, inspiration
	spiral: 10 mm slice thickness / 20 mm table feed (pitch 2:1) top to bottom scanning of the upper abdomen
Contrast media	i.a.: 60 ml non-ionic CM, iodine content: 300–320 mg/ml, mixed 1:1 with 60 ml NaCl solution (total volume: 120 ml) injection via intra-arterial catheter with tip in the superior mesenteric artery or splenic artery
Injection rate	2 ml/sec
Scan delay time	20 sec after start of bolus (early phase) 90 sec after start of bolus (late phase)
CT technique	120 kV, 250–350 mA, 512 matrix, inspiration
	1st spiral: 10 mm slice thickness / 10 mm table feed (pitch 1:1) bottom to top 2nd spiral: same location and parameters as 1st spiral
Reconstruction	4 mm interval, soft-tissue algorithm
Photography	12 on 1, patient information, scout view without and with cut lines, unenhanced series and both CM enhanced series at soft-tissue window from top to bottom, basal lung segments at lung window (with edge enhancement if necessary)
Remarks	1. CTAP is at present the most sensitive modality for pre-operative detection of liver lesions, but it is not suitable for lesion characterization (see liver protocol for lesion characterization, page 26). 2. Two scanning series are necessary since some perfusion defects in the early phase do not represent tumor tissue, but rather fatty areas, areas of reduced perfusion without pathologic relevance, or areas of reduced perfusion due to vessel compression by tumor. 3. If post-processing in 2D (multiplanar)/3D is required, the reconstruction interval should be 3 mm (approx. 30% of the nominal slice thickness). 4. The pitch can be increased up to 2:1.

Brief protocol
unenhanced
CM i.a.
60/60 ml
(CM/NaCl)
2 ml/sec
20/90 sec
10/10/4
bottom to top

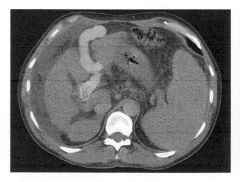 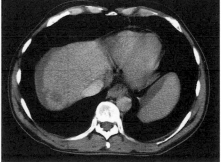

Injection of contrast agent via catheter in the superior mesenteric artery results in opacification of the reca-nalized umbilical vein with negligible enhancement of liver parenchyma. Pronounced liver cirrhosis and hepato-cellular carcinoma in the 7th liver segment (hypodense), splenomegaly, ascites.

Pancreas (pancreatitis, follow-up)

Region	above diaphragm to below uncinate process
Scout view	350 mm, 120 kV, 50–100 mA, pa
Unenhanced	120 kV, 75–150 mA, inspiration
	spiral: 10 mm slice thickness / 20 mm table feed (pitch 2:1) top to bottom scanning through the upper abdomen
Contrast media	i.v.: 100 ml non-ionic CM, iodine content: 300–320 mg/ml oral: 500 ml over 15 min (only if clinically acceptable), the last cup immediately before scanning
Injection rate	2.5 ml/sec
Scan delay time	40 sec after start of bolus
CT technique	120 kV, 175–300 mA, 512 matrix, inspiration
	1st spiral: 5 mm slice thickness / 5 mm table feed (pitch 1:1) bottom to top, entire pancreatic region (as determined on unenhanced scans) 2nd spiral: 10 mm slice thickness / 10 mm table feed (pitch 1:1) bottom to top, remainder of the liver to above diaphragm
Reconstruction	10 mm interval for unenhanced scan, soft-tissue algorithm 5 mm interval for 1st spiral, soft-tissue algorithm 8 mm interval for 2nd spiral, soft-tissue algorithm
Photography	12 on 1, patient information, scout view without and with cut lines, unenhanced scan at soft-tissue window from top to bottom, CM enhanced series at soft-tissue window from top to bottom, basal lung segments at lung window (with edge enhancement if necessary)
Remarks	1. Overlap last section of the 1st spiral with first section of the 2nd spiral. 2. Normal tap water or carbonated mineral water can be used as an alternative to positive (radiodense) oral contrast material. This will make the duodenal wall appear bright (CM enhancement) against the lumen. Administer oral CM only if clinically justifiable. 3. Instruct the patient to breathe deeply before scanning. 4. If post-processing in 2D (multiplanar)/3D is required, the reconstruction interval of the pancreas spiral should be 2 mm (approx. 30% of the nominal slice thickness). Use 3D protocol for assessment of vessel infiltration. 5. The pitch can be increased up to 1.5:1.

6. Enhancement as an expression of normal parenchymal perfusion can be quantified by comparing
   the pre- and post-contrast CT values in an ROI
   (region of interest) (typical values: post-contrast
   increase > 30 HU).
7. 1–2 single scans through the pelvis may be necessary, since severe forms of pancreatitis may
   be associated with free fluid accumulations in the
   pelvis.
8. For oral CM administration, see "General remarks",
   page IX.

unenhanced
CM oral, i.v.
100 ml,
2.5 ml/sec
40 sec
5/5/5, 10/10/8
bottom to top

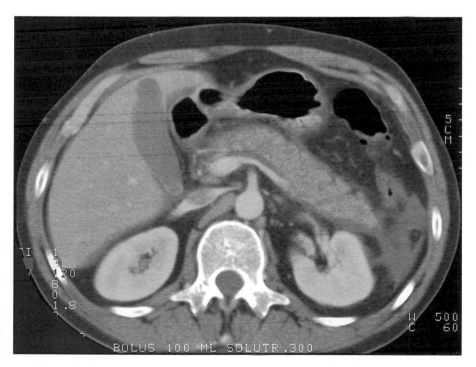

Exudative pancreatitis with fluid tunnels primarily in the area of the tail. The presence of complete parenchymal opacification excludes necrosis. Note the influx phenomenon in the inferior vena cava at the level of entrance of the renal vein.

Pancreas (tumor search, tumor staging, 3D reconstruction)

Region	above diaphragm to below uncinate process
Scout view	350 mm, 120 kV, 50–100 mA, pa
Unenhanced	120 kV, 75–150 mA, inspiration
	spiral: 10 mm slice thickness / 20 mm table feed (pitch 2:1) top to bottom scanning through expected pancreatic region
Contrast media	i.v.: 140 ml non-ionic CM, iodine content: 300–320 mg/ml oral: 500 ml over 15 min, the last cup immediately before scanning
Injection rate	4 ml/sec
Scan delay time	20 sec after start of bolus (arterial phase) 60 sec after start of bolus (parenchymal phase)
CT technique	120 kV, 175–300 mA, 512 matrix, inspiration
	1st spiral: 5 mm slice thickness / 5 mm table feed (pitch 1:1) bottom to top, entire pancreatic region (as determined on unenhanced scans) 2nd spiral: same location and parameters as 1st spiral 3rd spiral: 10 mm slice thickness / 10 mm table feed (pitch 1:1) bottom to top, remainder of the liver to above diaphragm
Reconstruction	10 mm interval for unenhanced scan, soft-tissue algorithm 3 mm interval for 1st and 2nd spiral, soft-tissue algorithm 8 mm interval for 3rd spiral, soft-tissue algorithm
Photography	12 on 1, patient information, scout view without and with cut lines, unenhanced scan and CM enhanced series at soft-tissue window from top to bottom, basal lung segments at lung window (with edge enhancement if necessary)
Remarks	1. Normal tap water or carbonated mineral water can be used as an alternative to positive (radiodense) oral contrast material. This will make the duodenal wall appear bright (CM enhancement) against the lumen. Administer oral CM only if clinically justifiable. 2. Two scanning series will detect both hyper- and hypovascularized lesions. 3. Instruct the patient to breathe deeply before scanning. 4. For post-processing in 2D (multiplanar)/3D, the reconstruction interval of the pancreas spiral should be 2 mm (approx. 30% of the nominal section thickness). Reconstruct both phases to visualize arterial or venous vascular infiltration.

Brief protocol
unenhanced CM oral, i.v. 140 ml 4 ml/sec 20/60 sec 5/5/3, 10/10/8 bottom to top

5. The pitch can be increased up to 1.5:1.
6. In selected cases, it might be advantageous to inject 10–20 mg Glucagon® intravenously for optimal duodenal distension.
7. For oral CM administration, see "General remarks", page IX.

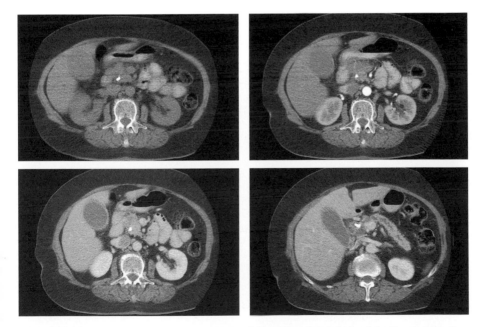

Sonographically suspected mass in the pancreatic head. Unenhanced study for localizing the pancreas. During the arterial phase, there is visualization of a filiform artery in a 1.8 cm tumor in the pancreatic head. The tumor appears hypodense compared to the CM enhanced parenchyma in the venous phase. Dilatation of the pancreatic and common bile duct after stent implantation.

Kidneys

Region	kidneys
Scout view	350 mm, 120 kV, 50–100 mA, pa
Unenhanced	120 kV, 50–125 mA, inspiration
	spiral: 10 mm slice thickness / 20 mm table feed (pitch 2:1) top to bottom scanning through expected kidney region
Contrast media	i.v.: 80 ml non-ionic CM, iodine content: 300–320 mg/ml oral: 1000 ml over 60 min
Injection rate	2 ml/sec
Scan delay time	40 sec after start of bolus
CT technique	120 kV, 75–250 mA, 512 matrix, inspiration
	spiral: 5 mm slice thickness / 5 mm table feed (pitch 1:1) bottom to top, both kidneys as determined on unenhanced scans
Reconstruction	5 mm interval, soft-tissue algorithm
Photography	12 on 1, patient information, scout view without and with cut lines, unenhanced and CM enhanced series at soft-tissue window from top to bottom
Remarks	1. With a caudo-cranial scanning direction, the scanning area can be extended cranially for evaluation of tumor extension and potential liver metastases.
	2. For assessment of suspected thrombosis of the renal vein or inferior vena cava in patients with known malignancy, the scan delay should be 70 sec and the scanning area should extend to the right atrium.
	3. For suspected renal artery stenosis, use the CT angiography protocol for the renal arteries without oral administration of contrast material.
	4. Instruct the patient to breathe deeply before scanning.
	5. Sagittal 2D reconstruction with a reconstruction interval of 2 mm (approx. 30% of the nominal slice thickness) is recommended for evaluation of tumor extension.
	6. The pitch can be increased up to 2:1.
	7. In case of a pathologic finding in the renal pelvis/ureter, delayed scanning with 100–150 mA after 5 min may be necessary. Alternatively, 20 ml contrast material for opacification of the renal pelvis/ureter may be administered about 5 min before scanning.

**unenhanced
CM oral, i.v.
80 ml
2 ml/sec
40 sec
5/5/5
bottom to top**

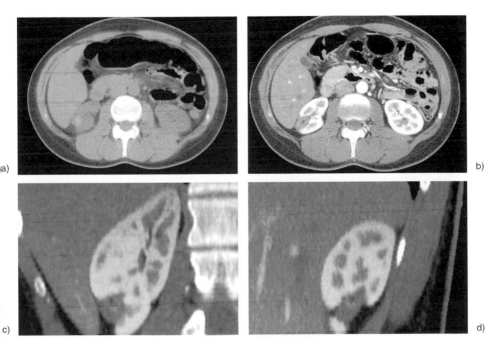

a)

b)

c)

d)

(a) + (b) 26-year-old female with sonographically unclear mass in the right kidney. Scans before and after intravenous administration of contrast material.
(c) + (d) Coronal and sagittal reconstruction of the contrast-enhanced series. The diagnosis of an angiomyolipoma is suggested by the absence of malignancy signs and the demonstration of fatty areas in the lesion.

Kidneys with abdomen and pelvis

Region	above diaphragm to pubic symphysis
Scout view	500 mm, 120 kV, 50–100 mA, pa
Unenhanced	120 kV, 50–125 mA, inspiration
	spiral: 10 mm slice thickness / 20 mm table feed (pitch 2:1) top to bottom scanning through expected kidney region
Contrast media	i.v.: 120 ml non-ionic CM, iodine content: 300–320 mg/ml oral: 1000 ml over 60 min rectal: 500 ml immediately before scanning
Injection rate	2.5 ml/sec
Scan delay time	40 sec after start of bolus
CT technique	120 kV, 175–300 mA, 512 matrix, inspiration
	1st spiral: 5 mm slice thickness / 5 mm table feed (pitch 1:1) bottom to top, both kidneys as determined on unenhanced scans 2nd spiral: 10 mm slice thickness / 10 mm table feed (pitch 1:1) bottom to top, remainder of the liver to above diaphragm 3rd spiral: 10 mm slice thickness / 10 mm table feed (pitch 1:1) bottom to top, symphysis to lower kidney pole
Reconstruction	5 mm interval for kidney spiral, soft-tissue algorithm 8 mm interval for 2nd and 3rd spiral, soft-tissue algorithm
Photography	12 on 1, patient information, scout view without and with cut lines, soft-tissue window from top to bottom, basal lung segments at lung window (with edge enhancement if necessary)
Remarks	1. Overlap one section between adjacent spirals.
	2. For assessment of suspected thrombosis of the renal vein or inferior vena cava in patients with known malignancy, the scan delay should be 70 sec and the scanning area should extend to the right atrium.
	3. For suspected renal artery stenosis, use the CT angiography protocol for the renal arteries without oral administration of contrast material.
	4. Have the patient drink a cup of water immediately before scanning for better filling of the stomach.
	5. Instruct the patient to breathe deeply before scanning.
	6. Sagittal 2D reconstruction with a reconstruction interval of 2 mm (approx. 30% of the nominal slice thickness) is recommended for evaluation of tumor extension. Use identical FOV and matrix for all spirals.

7. The pitch can be increased up to 2:1.
8. In case of a pathologic finding in the renal pelvis/ureter, delayed scanning with 150–200 mA after 5 min may be necessary. Alternatively, 20 ml contrast material for opacification of the renal pelvis/ureter may be administered about 5 min before scanning.
9. Co-administration of 20 mg metoclopramide (MCP) with the first cup of contrast material accelerates the CM passage.
10. For oral and rectal CM administration, see "General remarks", page IX.

**unenhanced
CM oral, rectal
i.v.
120 ml
2.5 ml/sec
40 sec
5/5/5, 10/10/8
bottom to top**

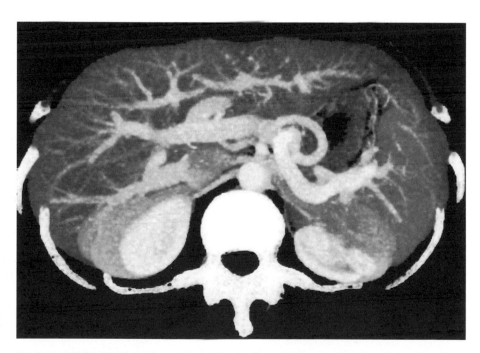

Cranio-caudal MIP of the first and second spiral showing the portal venous system, the splenic vein, and both renal arteries. Normal appearance of both venous systems; the renal artery stenosis on the left was confirmed by Doppler ultrasound.

Adrenal glands

Region	adrenals
Scout view	250 mm, 120 kV, 50–100 mA, pa
Unenhanced	120 kV, 75–150 mA, inspiration
	spiral: 5 mm slice thickness / 5 mm table feed (pitch 1:1) top to bottom scanning through expected adrenal region
Contrast media	i.v.: 120 ml non-ionic CM, iodine content: 300–320 mg/ml
Injection rate	2.5 ml/sec
Scan delay time	50 sec after start of bolus
CT technique	120 kV, 75–200 mA, inspiration
	spiral: 5 mm slice thickness / 5 mm table feed (pitch 1:1) top to bottom, only adrenals as determined on the unenhanced scans

Only for adrenal tumors (diameter > 2.5 cm)

Reconstruction	3 mm interval for pre-contrast scans and for CM enhanced series if required, soft-tissue algorithm, magnified reconstruction of scans containing adrenals (smaller FOV)
Photography	12 on 1, patient information, scout view without and with cut lines, unenhanced series, magnification, CM enhanced series if applicable, at soft-tissue window from top to bottom
Remarks	1. The risk of inducing a hypertensive crisis in patients with pheochromocytoma by intravenous administration of contrast material is discussed controversially in the literature. We recommend that phentolamine for intravenous injection (Regitin®) should be readily available for emergencies. 2. In patients with clinically suspected pheochromocytoma and no adrenal abnormalities, scanning should be extended to the area of the aortic bifurcation and, if necessary, to the urinary bladder after CM administration to exclude extra-adrenal localization (Zuckerkandl's organ). 3. The tube current should not exceed 75 mA in slender patients.

**unenhanced
CM i.v.
if required
120 ml
2.5 ml/sec
50 sec
5/5/3
top to bottom**

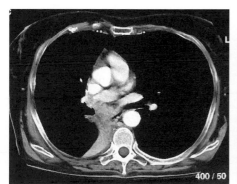 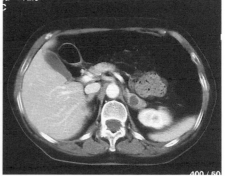

Central bronchogenic carcinoma on the right with a metastasis in the left adrenal. Intravenous administration of contrast material for delineation of the pulmonary tumor also improves visualization of the hypodense lesion in the left adrenal.

Paranasal sinuses

Region	posterior wall of sphenoidal sinuses to anterior wall of frontal sinuses
Scout view	200 mm, 120 kV, 50 mA, lateral
Contrast media	–
Injection rate	–
Scan delay time	–
CT technique	120 kV, 50–150 mA, 512 matrix
	patient in prone position with reclined head, gantry inclination perpendicular to orbital floor (coronal section)
	spiral: 5 mm slice thickness / 10 mm table feed (pitch 2:1) posterior to anterior
Reconstruction	5 mm interval, lung/bone algorithm
Photography	12 on 1, patient information, scout view without and with cut lines, soft-tissue window from posterior to anterior, bone window from posterior to anterior
Remarks	1. Since the lenses are in the scanning area, strict indication and minimal tube current (≤ 50 mA) are mandatory. A pitch of 2:1 further reduces the x-ray dose by a factor of 2.
	2. Use a 2 mm interval for multiplanar reconstruction of the data set in the axial direction.
	3. Multiple radiodense tooth fillings may produce artifacts in coronal sections and considerably impair interpretation. Such artifacts can be avoided by axial scanning with coronal reconstruction.
	4. For highly detailed resolution, we recommend a scan time of 2 sec and conventional, incremental scanning at a slice thickness of 5 mm.
	5. For pre-operative planning, the reconstruction interval in the area of the anterior ethmoidal cells (orifices!) may have to be changed to 3 mm.
	6. For tumor staging, an axial examination of the frontal skull and neck is recommended after 120 ml of i.v. CM, injection rate 2 ml/sec, 70 sec scan delay, 5/5/5, as well as coronal reconstruction in the area of the paranasal sinuses (with a reconstruction interval of 2 mm).

Brief protocol

unenhanced
5/10/5
coronal
low-dose
technique

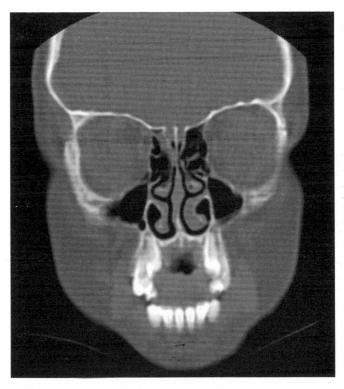

Coronal section through the paranasal sinuses. Sufficient delineation of the bony portions with patent orifices on both sides despite minimal energy (50 mA) and a pitch of 2:1 (corresponding to 25 mAs per section).

Dental CT (with multiplanar reconstruction)

Region	entire maxilla or mandible, depending on diagnostic problem
Scout view	150 mm, 120 kV, 50 mA, lateral
Contrast media	–
Injection rate	–
Scan delay time	–
CT technique	120 kV, 50 mA, 512 matrix, 2 sec scan time, 130 mm FOV
	patient in supine position with head fixed, gantry inclination parallel to the branch of jaw to be examined, place cellulose or a non-radiodense wedge between the teeth
	no spiral, 1.5 mm slice thickness / 1 mm table feed
Reconstruction	lung/bone algorithm
Postprocessing	multiplanar sectioning along the row of teeth, coronal (image similar to OPTG) and sagittal (perpendicular to branch of jaw)
Photography	patient information, scout view, 12 on 1 for coronal sections, 36 on 1 for sagittal sections, bone window
Remarks	1. The slice thickness should not be greater than 2 mm since partial volume effects may reduce the delineation of the mandibular canal and other structures.
	2. The energy per section should not exceed 100 mA.
	3. Securely fix the patient's head.

Brief protocol
unenhanced 1.5/1 axial, 50 mA multiplanar reconstruction coronal/sagittal

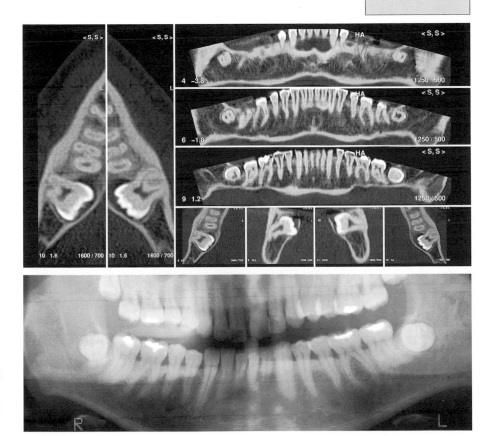

Status pre extraction of both transversely located third molars. Axial, coronal, and sagittal reconstructions. Matching OPTG.

CT angiography:
Thoracic aortic aneurysm (TAA)

Region	above clavicles to below diaphragm
Scout view	450 mm, 120 kV, 50–100 mA, pa
Contrast media	i.v.: 90 ml non-ionic CM, iodine content: 300–320 mg/ml
Injection rate	3 ml/sec
Scan delay time	20 sec after start of bolus
CT technique	120 kV, 100–175 mA, 512 matrix, inspiration
	spiral: 3 mm slice thickness / 5 mm table feed (pitch 1.7:1) bottom to top
Reconstruction	3 mm interval, soft-tissue algorithm
Postprocessing	multiplanar sectioning along the aorta, coronal and sagittal reconstructions, MIP or surface rendering
Photography	12 on 1, patient information, scout view without and with cut lines, axial sections (every 3rd section) at soft-tissue window, reconstructions (multiplanar, MIP, surface) in pertinent projections
Remarks	1. Use a reconstruction interval of 2 mm for post-processing.
	2. Depending on the surgical problem, visualization of the thoracic origins (intercostal arteries) may be important and requires selective reconstruction of the aorta from the raw data.
	3. Multiplanar reconstruction along a path does not require additional editing. Display several sections parallel to the path. Distance measurements represent true distances.
	4. MIP requires editing, e.g. removal of the vertebral column and ribs. This may be done section per section or along a path on the sagittal image. Separation of aortic calcifications may be difficult.
	5. 3D surface displays may be generated by editing or by establishment of a threshold value. Best pre-operative procedure for 3D display.
	6. Instruct the patient to breathe deeply before scanning and point out that smooth breathing is allowed in case of shortness of breath.

Brief protocol
CM i.v. 90 ml 3 ml/sec 20 sec 3/5/3 bottom to top

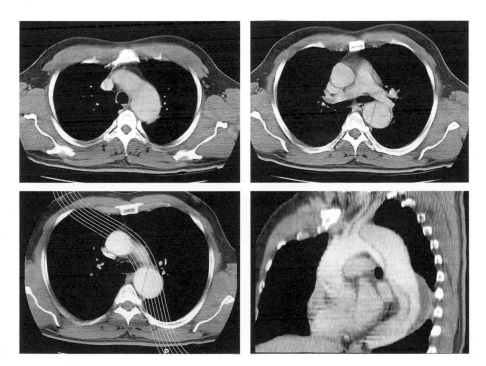

Dissecting thoracic aortic aneurysm, type III. Involvement of the origins of cranial vessels in this process remains unclear on axial scans. Multiplanar reconstruction along the aorta shows that these vessels arise from the true lumen.

CT angiography:
Abdominal aortic aneurysm (AAA)

Region	above diaphragm to level of hip joints
Scout view	450 mm, 120 kV, 50–100 mA, pa
Contrast media	i.v.: 100 ml non-ionic CM, iodine content: 300–320 mg/ml
Injection rate	3 ml/sec
Scan delay time	20 sec after start of bolus
CT technique	120 kV, 150–200 mA, 512 matrix, inspiration
	spiral: 5 mm slice thickness / 10 mm table feed (pitch 2:1)
	top to bottom
Reconstruction	5 mm interval, soft-tissue algorithm
Postprocessing	multiplanar sectioning along the aorta, coronal and sagittal reconstructions, MIP or surface rendering
Photography	12 on 1, patient information, scout view without and with cut lines, axial sections (every 2nd section) at soft-tissue window, reconstructions (multiplanar, MIP, surface) in pertinent projections
Remarks	1. Use a reconstruction interval of 3 mm for post-processing.
	2. Multiplanar reconstruction along a path does not require additional editing. Display several sections parallel to the path. Distance measurements represent true distances.
	3. MIP requires editing, e.g. removal of the vertebral column. This may be done section per section or along a path on the sagittal image. Separation of aortic calcifications may be difficult.
	4. 3D surface displays may be generated by editing or by establishment of a threshold value. Best pre-operative procedure for 3D display.
	5. Instruct the patient to breathe deeply before scanning and point out that smooth breathing is allowed in case of shortness of breath.
	6. Do not give oral contrast material (impairs identification of vessels on 3D images).

CM i.v.
100 ml
3 ml/sec
20 sec
5/10/5
top to bottom

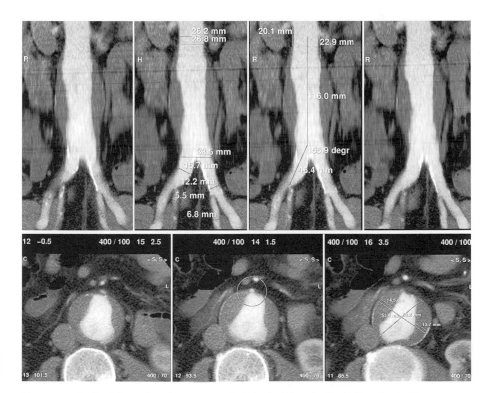

Measurements of an infrarenal aortic aneurysm prior to implantation of a Stentor® prosthesis. Homogeneous opacification of the entire aorta; circle shows origin of the inferior mesenteric artery.

CT angiography:
Thoracic and abdominal aortic aneurysm

Region	above clavicles to level of hip joints
Scout view	600 mm, 120 kV, 50–100 mA, pa
Contrast media	i.v.: 140 ml non-ionic CM, iodine content: 300–320 mg/ml
Injection rate	3 ml/sec
Scan delay time	20 sec after start of bolus
CT technique	120 kV, 100–250 mA, 512 matrix, inspiration
	spiral: 5 mm slice thickness / 10 mm table feed (pitch 2:1) top to bottom, entire aorta with one spiral
Reconstruction	5 mm interval, soft-tissue algorithm
Postprocessing	multiplanar sectioning along the aorta, coronal and sagittal reconstructions, MIP or surface rendering
Photography	12 on 1, patient information, scout view without and with cut lines, axial sections (every 2nd section) at soft-tissue window, reconstructions (multiplanar, MIP, surface) in pertinent projections
Remarks	1. Shallow breathing minimally affects image quality in the pelvic area. One continuous spiral is preferable to several spirals for uninterrupted reconstruction.
	2. Use a reconstruction interval of 3 mm for post-processing.
	3. For assessing the extent of dissection and involvement of aortic branches such as cranial vessels, renal arteries or mesenteric arteries, these areas should be scanned with a 2nd spiral at a slice thickness of 3 mm and a variable pitch (1:1 to 2:1) during breath-hold. Give second contrast bolus of 60 ml, 2 ml/sec, scan delay 25 sec; reconstruction interval of 1 mm for multiplanar reconstruction.
	4. Multiplanar reconstruction along a path does not require additional editing. Display several sections parallel to the path. Distance measurements represent true distances.
	5. MIP requires editing, e.g. removal of the vertebral column and ribs. This may be done section per section or along a path on the sagittal image. Separation of aortic calcifications may be difficult.
	6. 3D surface displays may be generated by editing or by establishment of a threshold value. Best pre-operative procedure for 3D display.

7. Instruct the patient to breathe deeply before scanning and point out that smooth breathing is allowed in case of shortness of breath.

CM i.v.
140 ml
3 ml/sec
20 sec
5/10/5
top to bottom

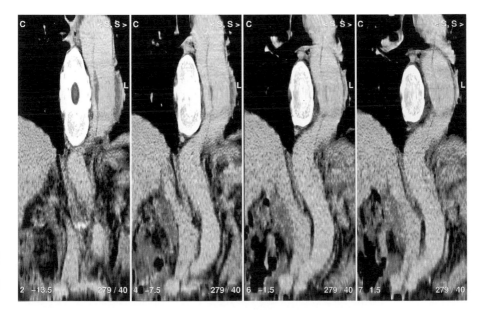

Dissecting thoracic aortic aneurysm with infrarenal extension. Multiplanar reconstruction along the aorta with distortion of surrounding structures.

CT angiography:
Renal arteries

Region	renal arteries
Scout view	350 mm, 120 kV, 50–100 mA, pa
Unenhanced	120 kV, 50–125 mA, inspiration
	spiral: 10 mm slice thickness / 20 mm table feed (pitch 2:1) top to bottom scanning through expected kidney region
Contrast media	i.v.: 90 ml non-ionic CM, iodine content: 300–320 mg/ml
Injection rate	3 ml/sec
Scan delay time	25 sec after start of bolus
CT technique	120 kV, 75–250 mA, 512 matrix, inspiration
	spiral: 3 mm slice thickness / 3 mm table feed (pitch 1:1) top to bottom, only area of the renal arteries as determined on the unenhanced scans. The origin of the renal arteries should be in the upper third of the spiral (descending course of the arteries)
Reconstruction	1 mm interval, soft-tissue algorithm
Postprocessing	multiplanar sectioning along the renal arteries, coronal and axial reconstructions, MIP or surface rendering
Photography	12 on 1, patient information, scout view without and with cut lines, axial sections (every 3rd section) at soft-tissue window, reconstructions (multiplanar, MIP, surface) in pertinent projections
Remarks	1. Multiplanar reconstruction along a path does not require additional editing. Display several sections parallel to the path. Distance measurements represent true distances.
	2. MIP requires editing, e.g. removal of the vertebral column. This may be done section per section or along a path on the sagittal image. Separation of aortic calcifications may be difficult.
	3. 3D surface displays may be generated by editing or by establishment of a threshold value. Note: the former bears the risk of misinterpretation of anatomical structures, the latter cannot differentiate partial volume effects from true density values which may lead to over- or underestimation of stenoses or even creation of pseudostenoses.
	4. Instruct the patient to breathe deeply before scanning.
	5. Reduction of the slice thickness to 2 or 1 mm will increase resolution along the z-axis. Most tubes have a maximal capacity of only 150 mA when a small

Brief protocol
unenhanced **CM i.v.** **90 ml** **3 ml/sec** **25 sec** **3/3/1** **top to bottom**

focus is used, which increases image noise and thus impairs image quality. Soft filters compensate for noise at the expense of spatial resolution.

6. The pitch can be increased up to 2:1.

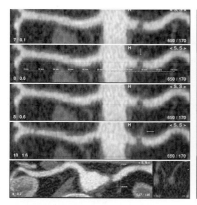

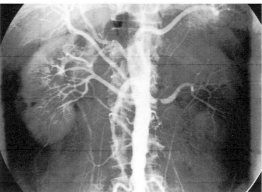

57-year-old patient (85 kg, 175 cm) with hypertension of unknown etiology. Filiform renal artery stenosis on the left, adrenal artery arising from the stenotic area (arrow). Findings corresponding to those obtained by digital subtraction angiography.

Cardiac CT (with multiplanar reconstruction)

Region	aortic arch to apex of heart
Scout view	350 mm, 120 kV, 50–100 mA, lateral
Contrast media	i.v.: 60 ml non-ionic CM, iodine content: 300–320 mg/ml
Injection rate	2.5 ml/sec
Scan delay time	30 sec after start of bolus
CT technique	120 kV, 125–200 mA, 512 matrix, inspiration maximal gantry inclination parallel to the long heart axis spiral: 10 mm slice thickness / 10 mm table feed (pitch 1:1) bottom to top, entire heart region
Reconstruction	5 mm interval, soft-tissue algorithm (without post-processing) 3 mm interval, soft-tissue algorithm (for post-processing)
Postprocessing	multiplanar sectioning along the long heart axis every 3 mm, corresponding to a coronal heart section
Photography	12 on 1, patient information, scout view without and with cut lines, 5 mm original scans and reconstructions at soft-tissue window, original scans at lung window (with edge enhancement if required)
Remarks	1. To facilitate evaluation, axial sections can be calculated from the original data by multiplanar reconstruction. 2. Increase scan delay to 40 sec in patients with known heart failure. 3. Reduction of the table feed and slice thickness, e.g. 5/5/5, does not improve image quality, since image quality will be affected by more heart beats. Alternatively, a spiral with 5 mm slice thickness and 10 mm table feed can be used (pitch 2:1). 4. Instruct the patient to breathe deeply before scanning.

Brief protocol

CM i.v.
60 ml
2.5 ml/sec
30 sec
10/10/5
bottom to top

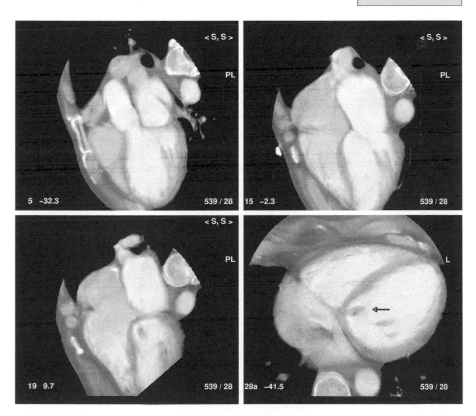

Multiplanar reconstruction of the heart. Visualization of an intracardiac thrombus of 1.6 cm in diameter (arrow). Normal appearance of anterior and posterior papillary muscle. The section planes are along the long and short heart axis.

Short-spiral CT

Abdomen and pelvis

Region	above diaphragm to pubic symphysis
Scout view	512 mm, 120 kV, 50–100 mA, pa
Contrast media	i.v.: 120 ml non-ionic CM, iodine content: 300–320 mg/ml oral: 1000 ml over 60 min rectal: 500 ml immediately before scanning
Injection rate	2.5 ml/sec
Scan delay time	50 sec after start of bolus
CT technique	120 kV, 165–290 mA, 512 matrix, inspiration spiral: 24–32 rotations 8 mm slice thickness / 8 mm table feed (pitch 1:1) top to bottom, followed by incremental: dynamic screening 8 mm slice thickness / 8 mm table feed to symphysis, breaks for breathing
Reconstruction	8 mm interval, standard algorithm
Photography	12 on 1, patient information, scout view without and with cut lines, soft-tissue window from top to bottom, basal lung segments at lung window
Remarks	1. Have the patient drink a cup of water immediately before scanning for better filling of the stomach. 2. Instruct the patient to breathe deeply before scanning. 3. If post-processing in 2D (multiplanar)/3D is required, the reconstruction interval should be 3 mm (approx. 30% of the nominal slice thickness). 4. The table feed can be increased up to 16 mm (pitch 2:1). 5. In case of a pathologic finding in the kidneys, ureters, or bladder, delayed scanning with 165–210 mA after 5 min may be necessary. 6. Rectal CM administration should be performed for all gynecological examinations and suspected pathology in the colon/rectum. As an alternative to a contrast enema, a pre-packaged implementation device (approx. 150 ml) can be used. 7. Co-administration of 20 mg metoclopramide (MCP) with the first cup of contrast material accelerates the CM passage. 8. For oral and rectal CM administration, see "General remarks", page IX.

Brief protocol
CM oral, rectal
i.v.
120 ml
2.5 ml/sec
50 sec
8/8/8
top to bottom

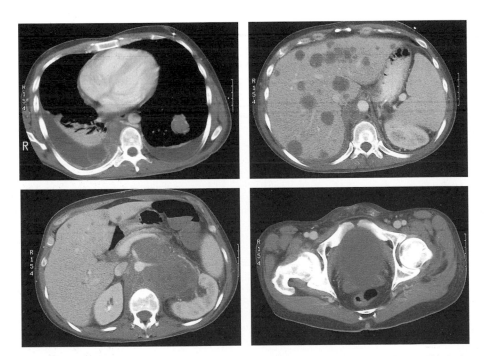

Testicular germ cell tumor. Intrapulmonary metastasis in the left lower lobe (first section of the spiral), multiple cystic and necrotic liver metastases in all segments, massive bulky lymphoma in the retrocrural and retroperitoneal area with complete encasement of the left renal artery (delayed contrast enhancement of the renal parenchyma) and of the superior mesenteric artery. No inguinal lymphadenopathy. Sufficient opacification of the iliac and femoral vessels also at the end of the incremental scan series.

Chest and upper abdomen

Region	above clavicles to lower kidney pole
Scout view	512 mm, 120 kV, 50–100 mA, pa
Contrast media	i.v.: 120 ml (abdomen) + 30 ml (chest) non-ionic CM, iodine content: 300–320 mg/ml oral: 1000 ml over 60 min
Injection rate	2.5 ml/sec for abdomen, 2 ml/sec for chest bolus
Scan delay time	50 sec after start of bolus for abdominal spiral 15 sec after start of bolus for chest spiral
CT technique	120 kV, 110–290 mA, 512 matrix, inspiration 1st spiral: 24–32 rotations 8 mm slice thickness / 8 mm table feed (pitch 1:1) top to bottom, liver, starting above diaphragm incremental: autosequence 8 mm slice thickness / 8 mm table feed to lower kidney pole start chest bolus 2nd spiral: 24–32 rotations 8 mm slice thickness / 8 mm table feed (pitch 1:1) or measure chest distance on scout view and adjust table feed to cover entire chest with one spiral (pitch ≥ 1:1) top to bottom in case of incomplete chest examination: incremental: dynamic screening 8 mm slice thickness / 8 mm table feed remainder of the lung to below both sinuses (or to below adrenals), breaks for breathing
Reconstruction	8 mm interval for 1st spiral, standard algorithm 8 mm interval for 2nd spiral, lung/bone algorithm
Photography	12 on 1, patient information, scout view without and with cut lines, soft-tissue window from top to bottom, lung window

Brief protocol
CM oral, i.v.
120/30 ml
2.5/2 ml/sec
50/15 sec
8/8/8
top to bottom

Remarks

1. Overlap one scan between adjacent spirals.
2. Have the patient drink a cup of water immediately before scanning for better filling of the stomach.
3. Instruct the patient to breathe deeply before scanning.
4. A suitable contrast agent for the esophagus is Esopho-Cat® (2 tablespoons immediately before scanning).
5. If post-processing in 2D (multiplanar)/3D is required, the reconstruction interval should be 3 mm (approx. 30% of the nominal slice thickness), use identical FOV and matrix for both spirals.
6. The table feed can be increased up to 16 mm (pitch 2:1).
7. In case of a pathologic finding in the renal pelvis/ureter, delayed scanning after 5 min may be necessary.
8. For oral CM administration, see "General remarks", page IX.

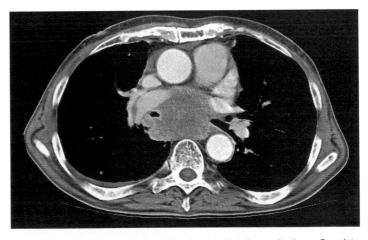

Extensive bronchogenic carcinoma infiltrating the posterior mediastinum. Complete opacification of all vessels is necessary to demonstrate potential vessel infiltration.

Neck and chest

Region	below base of skull to below both sinuses of diaphragm include adrenals in bronchogenic carcinoma
Scout view	chest: 512 mm, 120 kV, 50–100 mA, pa neck: 256 mm, 120 kV, 50–100 mA, lateral
Contrast media	i.v.: 80 ml (chest) + 40 ml (neck) non-ionic CM, iodine content: 300–320 mg/ml
Injection rate	2 ml/sec for chest and neck bolus
Scan delay time	30 sec after start of chest bolus, 20 sec after start of neck bolus
CT technique	120 kV, 110–220 mA, inspiration

1st spiral: 24–32 rotations
8 mm slice thickness / 8 mm table feed (pitch 1:1), or
measure chest distance on scout view and adjust table feed
to cover entire chest with one spiral (pitch ≥1:1)
top to bottom

in case of incomplete chest examination:

incremental: dynamic screening
8 mm slice thickness / 8 mm table feed
remainder of the lung to below both sinuses (or to below both
adrenals), breaks for breathing

reposition patient with arms parallel to trunk, angle gantry parallel to the inter-
vertebral disc C4–C5, start neck bolus

2nd spiral: 24 rotations
5 mm slice thickness / 5 mm table feed (pitch 1:1)
top to bottom

Reconstruction	8 mm interval for 1st spiral, lung/bone algorithm 5 mm interval for 2nd spiral, standard algorithm
Photography	12 on 1, patient information, scout view without and with cut lines, soft-tis- sue window from top to bottom, lung window from top to bottom
Remarks	1. A suitable contrast agent for the esophagus is Esopho-Cat® (2 tablespoons immediately before scanning). 2. If post-processing in 2D (multiplanar)/3D is required, the reconstruction inter- val should be 3 mm (approx. 30% of the nominal slice thickness).

Brief protocol

3. The table feed can be increased up to 16 mm (lung)/10 mm (neck) (pitch 2:1).
4. Edge enhancement (implemented in most scanners as a post-processing function) facilitates the detection of very small lung lesions.
5. Follow-up of intrapulmonary nodules during therapy may be done without intravenous administration of contrast material.
6. The tube current should not exceed 110 mA in slender patients.

CM i.v.
80/40 ml
2 ml/sec
30/20 sec
8/8/8, 5/5/5
top to bottom

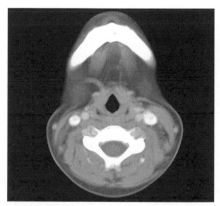 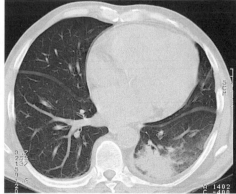

Indication: fever, questionable swelling of the neck lymph nodes, abnormal auscultation finding over the left lung. Normal appearance of the neck area with opacification of arteries and veins. Pneumonic infiltrate in the lower lobe of the left lung.

Chest, abdomen, and pelvis

Region	above clavicles to pubic symphysis
Scout view	512 mm, 120 kV, 50–100 mA, pa
Contrast media	i.v.: 120 ml (abdomen and pelvis) + 40 ml (chest) non-ionic CM, iodine content: 300–320 mg/ml oral: 1000 ml over 60 min rectal: 500 ml immediately before scanning
Injection rate	2.5 ml/sec for abdomen and pelvis, 2 ml/sec for chest bolus
Scan delay time	50 sec after start of bolus, 20 sec after start of chest bolus
CT technique	120 kV, 110–290 mA, 512 matrix, inspiration 1st spiral: 24–32 rotations 8 mm slice thickness / 8 mm table feed (pitch 1:1) top to bottom, liver, starting above diaphragm incremental: dynamic sequence 8 mm slice thickness / 8 mm table feed to symphysis, breaks for breathing start chest bolus 2nd spiral: 24–32 rotations 8 mm slice thickness / 8 mm table feed (pitch 1:1), or measure chest distance on scout view and adjust table feed to cover entire chest with one spiral (pitch ≥ 1:1) top to bottom in case of incomplete chest examination: incremental: dynamic screening 8 mm slice thickness / 8 mm table feed remainder of the lung to where first spiral started, breaks for breathing
Reconstruction	8 mm interval for 1st spiral, standard algorithm 8 mm interval for 2nd spiral, standard algorithm
Photography	12 on 1, patient information, scout view without and with cut lines, soft-tissue window from top to bottom, lung window
Remarks	1. Have the patient drink a cup of water immediately before scanning for better filling of the stomach.

Brief protocol
CM oral, rectal
i.v.
120/40 ml
2.5/2 ml/sec
50/20 sec
8/8/8
top to bottom

2. In case of a pathologic finding in the kidneys, ureters, or bladder, delayed scanning after 5 min may be necessary.
3. Rectal CM administration should be performed for all gynecological examinations and suspected pathology in the colon/rectum. As an alternative to a contrast enema, a pre-packaged implementation device (approx. 150 ml) can be used.
4. Co-administration of 20 mg metoclopramide (MCP) with the first cup of contrast material accelerates the CM passage.
5. A separate examination of the chest and abdomen/pelvis is recommended for fine assessment.

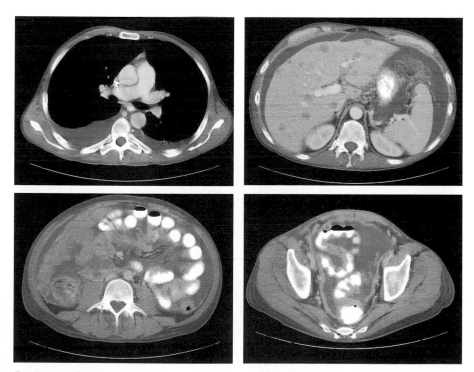

Excellent opacification of the thoracic vessels by the second bolus for the chest spiral. Liver scanning during the portal venous phase for demonstration of hypovascular metastases. Oral and rectal administration of contrast material for clearcut differentiation of bowel loops from tumor masses in peritoneal carcinomatosis.

Neck, chest, abdomen, and pelvis

Region	below base of skull to pubic symphysis
Scout view	512 mm, 120 kV, 50–100 mA, pa, set upper limit to base of skull
Contrast media	i.v.: 110 ml (abdomen and pelvis) + 40 ml (chest) + 30 ml (neck) non-ionic CM, iodine content: 300–320 mg/ml oral: 1000 ml over 60 min rectal: 500 ml immediately before scanning
Injection rate	2.5 ml/sec for abdomen and pelvis, 2 ml/sec for chest bolus 1.5 ml/sec for neck bolus
Scan delay time	50 sec after start of bolus, 20 sec after start of chest bolus 15 sec after start of neck bolus
CT technique	120 kV, 165–290 mA, 512 matrix, inspiration
	1st spiral: 24–32 rotations 8 mm slice thickness / 8 mm table feed (pitch 1:1) top to bottom, liver, starting above diaphragm
	incremental: dynamic sequence 8 mm slice thickness / 8 mm table feed to symphysis, breaks for breathing
	start chest bolus
	2nd spiral: 24–32 rotations 8 mm slice thickness / 8 mm table feed (pitch 1:1) or measure chest distance on scout view and adjust table feed to cover entire chest with one spiral (pitch ≥ 1:1) top to bottom
	in case of incomplete chest examination:
	incremental: dynamic screening 8 mm slice thickness / 8 mm table feed remainder of the lung to where 1st spiral started, breaks for breathing
	reposition patient's arms, start neck bolus
	3rd spiral: 24–32 rotations 5 mm slice thickness / 5 mm table feed (pitch 1:1) top to bottom, base of skull to where chest spiral started
Reconstruction	8 mm interval for 1st spiral, standard algorithm 8 mm interval for 2nd spiral, lung/bone algorithm 5 mm interval for 3rd spiral, standard algorithm

		Brief protocol

Photography — 12 on 1, patient information, scout view without and with cut lines, soft-tissue window from top to bottom, lung window

**CM oral, rectal
i.v.
110/40/30 ml
2.5/2/1.5 ml/sec
50/20/15 sec
8/8/8, 5/5/5
top to bottom**

Remarks

1. Since the chest and abdomen bolus may obscure neck pathology (tumors), we recommend to examine the neck or chest/neck separately from the abdomen/pelvis (at least 6 hours apart).
2. Overlap one scan between adjacent spirals.
3. Have the patient drink a cup of water immediately before scanning for better filling of the stomach.
4. Instruct the patient to breathe deeply before scanning.
5. If post-processing in 2D (multiplanar)/3D is required, the reconstruction interval should be 3 mm (approx. 30% of the nominal slice thickness).
7. In case of a pathologic finding in the kidneys, ureters, or bladder, delayed scanning after 5 min may be necessary.
8. Co-administration of 20 mg metoclopramide (MCP) with the first cup of contrast material accelerates the CM passage.
9. Rectal CM administration should be performed for all gynecological examinations and suspected pathology in the colon/rectum. As an alternative to a contrast enema, a pre-packaged implementation device (approx. 150 ml) can be used.

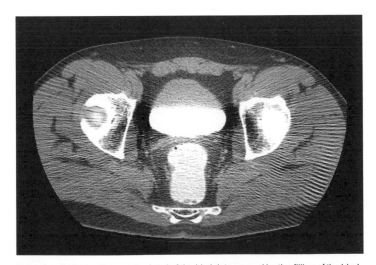

Beam-hardening artifacts at the level of the hip joints caused by the filling of the bladder with contrast material. Since the areas lateral to the bladder on both sides are nearly void of image information, pathology in these areas may escape detection.

Neck

Region	below base of skull to tip of lung or to above aortic arch if required
Scout view	256 mm, 120 kV, 50–100 mA, lateral
Contrast media	i.v.: 80 ml non-ionic CM, iodine content: 300–320 mg/ml
Injection rate	2 ml/sec
Scan delay time	40 sec after start of bolus
CT technique	120 kV, 65–165 mA matrix, inspiration incline gantry parallel to intervertebral disc C4–C5 spiral: 24–32 rotations 5 mm slice thickness / 5 mm table feed (pitch 1:1) top to bottom
Reconstruction	5 mm interval, standard algorithm
Photography	12 on 1, patient information, scout view without and with cut lines, soft-tissue window from top to bottom, scans containing lung segments at lung window from top to bottom
Remarks	1. For assessment of tumor extension (but not for lymph node staging), the scan delay may be increased to 70 sec and the amount of CM should be 120 ml. 2. Ask the patient not to swallow during the examination. 3. If post-processing in 2D (multiplanar)/3D is required, the reconstruction interval should be 2 mm (approx. 30% of the nominal slice thickness). 4. The table feed can be increased up to 10 mm (pitch 2:1). 5. The tube current should not be greater than 65 mA in patients with a slender neck.

Brief protocol

CM i.v.
80 ml
2 ml/sec
40 sec
5/5/5
top to bottom

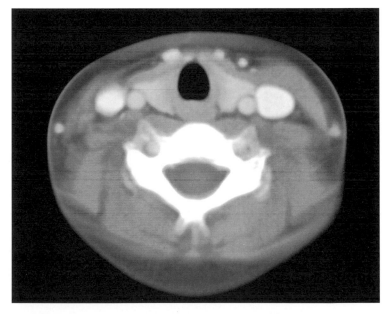

Normal appearance. Transverse section through the neck at the level of the thyroid with good opacification of arteries and veins and pronounced enhancement of the thyroid.

Chest

Region	above clavicles to below both sinuses of diaphragm include adrenals in bronchogenic carcinoma
Scout view	256 mm, 120 kV, 50–100 mA, pa
Contrast media	i.v.: 80 ml non-ionic CM, iodine content: 300–320 mg/ml
Injection rate	2 ml/sec
Scan delay time	30 sec after start of bolus
CT technique	120 kV, 110–210 mA, inspiration spiral: 24–32 rotations 8 mm slice thickness / 8 mm table feed (pitch 1:1), or measure chest distance on scout view and adjust table feed to cover entire chest with one spiral (pitch ≥ 1:1) top to bottom in case of incomplete chest examination: incremental: dynamic screening 8 mm slice thickness / 8 mm table feed remainder of the lung to below both sinuses (or to below both adrenals), breaks for breathing
Reconstruction	4 mm interval, lung/bone algorithm
Photography	12 on 1, patient information, scout view without and with cut lines, soft-tissue window from top to bottom, lung window from top to bottom (with additional edge enhancement if necessary)
Remarks	1. A suitable contrast agent for the esophagus is Esopho-Cat® (2 tablespoons immediately before scanning). 2. The reconstruction interval is 4 mm. To keep the number of images to be interpreted within reasonable limits, only alternate images should be photographed (corresponding to a reconstruction interval of 8 mm). In all unclear cases or if a CT scanner with a cine mode is available, the lung can be "leafed through" at the console. 3. For indications without search for intrapulmonary nodules smaller than 3 mm, the primary reconstruction interval can be increased to 8 mm. 4. The table feed can be increased up to 16 mm (pitch 2:1). 5. Edge enhancement (implemented in most scanners as a post-processing function) facilitates the detection of very small lung lesions.

Brief protocol

6. If post-processing in 2D (multiplanar)/3D is required, the reconstruction interval should be 3 mm (approx. 30% of the nominal slice thickness).
7. Follow-up of intrapulmonary nodules during therapy may be done without intravenous administration of contrast material.
8. The tube current should be reduced to a minimum in slender patients.

CM i.v.
80 ml
2 ml/sec
30 sec
8/8/4
top to bottom

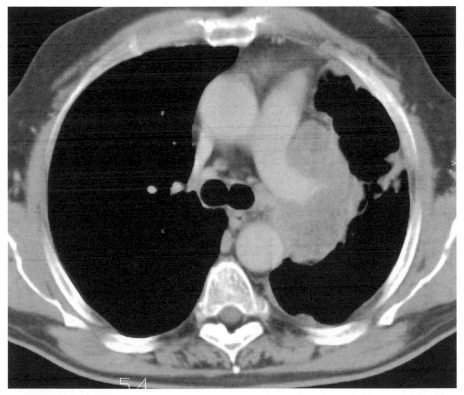

Central bronchogenic carcinoma. Optimal opacification of all thoracic vessels is necessary to assess vascular infiltration and mediastinal lymphadenopathy.

Chest in HR technique (high-resolution technique)

Region	tip of lung to below both sinuses of diaphragm
Scout view	256 mm, 120 kV, 50–100 mA, pa
Contrast media	–
Injection rate	–
Scan delay time	–
CT technique	137 kV, 110–220 mA, 512 matrix, 1–2 sec scan time, inspiration
	1–2 mm slice thickness / 10 mm table feed top to bottom, allow patient to breathe after 3–5 scans (≈20 sec)
Reconstruction	lung/bone algorithm
Photography	12 on 1, patient information, scout view without and with cut lines, soft-tissue window, lung window
Remarks	1. This protocol can only be used for assessing interstitial pulmonary changes or bronchiectasis. The 8–9 mm interscan gap limits the assessment of mediastinal lymphadenopathy or intrapulmonary nodules. 2. If contrast enhanced scans are required, use chest protocol in spiral technique. 3. If subpleurally increased interstitial reticulation (basal/dorsal) is noted, turn patient to prone position and acquire single scans through this area after 5 min (thereby excluding purely orthostatic changes). 4. With a scan time of 2 sec per section, more raw data can be acquired than with 1-sec scans, which improves contrast and resolution of details. 5. The tube current should not exceed 65 mA in slender patients.

Brief protocol

unenhanced
1–2/10
top to bottom

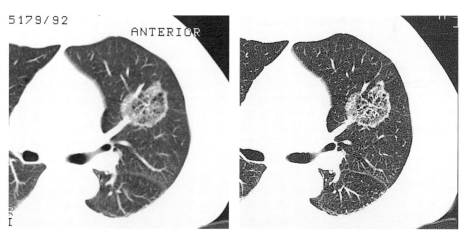

Differences between spiral CT and thin-section HR-CT. More detailed visualization of the pulmonary framework on the HR-CT scan. The infiltrate in the left upper lobe had disappeared at follow-up, 4 weeks later.

Upper abdomen

Region	above diaphragm to lower kidney pole
Scout view	256 mm, 120 kV, 50–100 mA, pa
Contrast media	i.v.: 120 ml non-ionic CM, iodine content: 300–320 mg/ml oral: 1000 ml over 60 min
Injection rate	2.5 ml/sec
Scan delay time	50 sec after start of bolus
CT technique	120 kV, 165–290 mA, 512 matrix, inspiration spiral: 24–32 rotations 8 mm slice thickness / 8 mm table feed (pitch 1:1) top to bottom incremental: autosequence 8 mm slice thickness / 8 mm table feed to lower kidney pole
Reconstruction	8 mm interval, standard algorithm
Photography	12 on 1, patient information, scout view without and with cut lines, soft-tissue window from top to bottom, basal lung segments at lung window
Remarks	1. Have the patient drink a cup of water immediately before scanning for better filling of the stomach. 2. Instruct the patient to breathe deeply before scanning. 3. If post-processing in 2D (multiplanar)/3D is required, the reconstruction interval should be 3 mm (approx. 30% of the nominal slice thickness). 4. The table feed can be increased up to 16 mm (pitch 2:1). 5. In case of a pathologic finding in the renal pelvis/ureter, delayed scanning after 5 min may be necessary. 6. For oral CM administration, see "General remarks", page IX.

Brief protocol
CM oral, i.v.
120 ml
2.5 ml/sec
50 sec
8/8/8
top to bottom

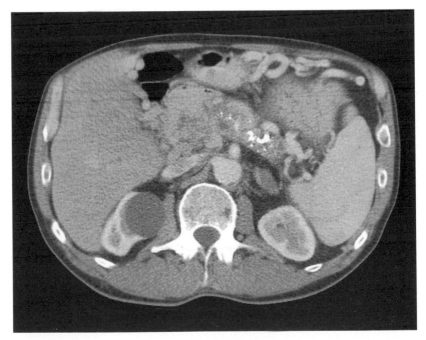

Chronic calcifying pancreatitis, early liver cirrhosis with portal hypertension, cavernous transformation of the portal vein and splenic vein thrombosis. Good opacification of collaterals along the greater curvature. Accessory finding: adrenal adenoma on the left, renal cyst on the right.

Pelvis

Region	lower kidney pole to pubic symphysis
Scout view	256 mm, 120 kV, 50–100 mA, pa
Contrast media	i.v.: 120 ml non-ionic CM, iodine content: 300–320 mg/ml oral: 1000 ml over 60 min rectal: 500 ml immediately before scanning
Injection rate	2.5 ml/sec
Scan delay time	70 sec after start of bolus
CT technique	120 kV, 165–290 mA, 512 matrix, inspiration spiral: 24–32 rotations 8 mm slice thickness / 8 mm table feed (pitch 1:1) top to bottom
Reconstruction	8 mm interval, standard algorithm
Photography	12 on 1, patient information, scout view without and with cut lines, soft-tissue window from top to bottom
Remarks	1. Beam-hardening artifacts at the level of the hip joints when the bladder is filled with contrast material make it very difficult to assess the pelvic wall in suspected lymphadenopathy. 2. Acquire delayed scans with CM filled bladder only for assessment of bladder pathology. 3. For assessment of suspected pelvic vein thrombosis, the scan delay should be at least 120 sec, and the injection rate should be reduced to 1.5 ml/sec. 4. If post-processing in 2D (multiplanar)/3D is required, the reconstruction interval of the spiral should be 3 mm (approx. 30% of the nominal slice thickness). 5. The table feed can be increased up to 16 mm (pitch 2:1). 6. Minimize energy (< 165 mA) especially in younger patients! 7. Always administer contrast material rectally. As an alternative to a contrast enema, a pre-packaged implementation device (approx. 150 ml) can be used. 8. Co-administration of 20 mg metoclopramide (MCP) with the first cup of contrast material accelerates the CM passage. 9. For oral and rectal CM administration, see "General remarks", page IX.

Brief protocol
CM oral, rectal
i.v.
120 ml
2.5 ml/sec
70 sec
8/8/8
top to bottom

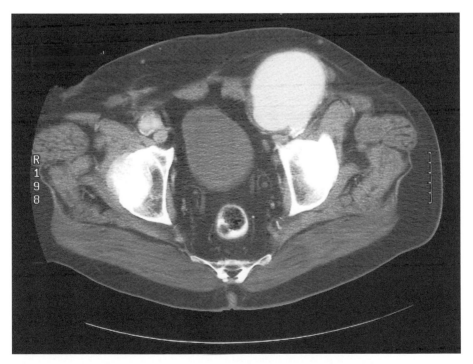

Pulsating tumor in the left groin after angiography. 7 cm false aneurysm of the femoral artery.

Liver (search for lesions of unknown origin)

Region	entire liver
Scout view	256 mm, 120 kV, 50–100 mA, pa
Unenhanced	120 kV, 110 mA, inspiration
	spiral: 24–32 rotations 8 mm slice thickness / 10 mm table feed (pitch 1.25:1) top to bottom
Contrast media	i.v.: 120 ml non-ionic CM, iodine content: 300–320 mg/ml oral: 1000 ml over 60 min
Injection rate	2.5 ml/sec
Scan delay time	60 sec after start of bolus (portal venous phase)
CT technique	120 kV, 165–290 mA, 512 matrix, inspiration
	spiral: 24–32 rotations 8 mm slice thickness / 8 mm table feed (pitch 1:1) bottom to top
Reconstruction	8 mm interval for unenhanced scan, standard algorithm 4 mm interval for CM enhanced series, standard algorithm
Photography	12 on 1, patient information, scout view without and with cut lines, unenhanced (every image) and enhanced series (every 2nd image) at soft-tissue window from top to bottom, basal lung segments after CM at lung window
Remarks	1. Two scanning series through the liver, unenhanced and during the portal venous phase, will detect both hypervascularized and hypovascularized metastases such as metastases from renal cell carcinoma, melanoma, breast cancer, and metastases from endocrine tumors. Small HCCs may also be hypervascularized; they are delineated on unenhanced images, and are nearly isodense to liver parenchyma during the portal venous phase. 2. The reconstruction interval is 4 mm. To keep the number of images to be interpreted within reasonable limits, only alternate images of the post-contrast series should be photographed (corresponding to a reconstruction interval of 8 mm). In all unclear cases or if a CT scanner with a cine mode is available, the liver can be "leafed through" at the console. 3. If post-processsing in 2D (multiplanar)/3D is required, the reconstruction interval should be 3 mm (approx. 30% of the nominal slice thickness).

Brief protocol

**unenhanced
CM oral, i.v.
120 ml
2.5 ml/sec
60 sec
8/8/4
bottom to top**

4. The table feed can be increased up to 16 mm (pitch 2:1).
5. For oral CM administration, see "General remarks", page IX.

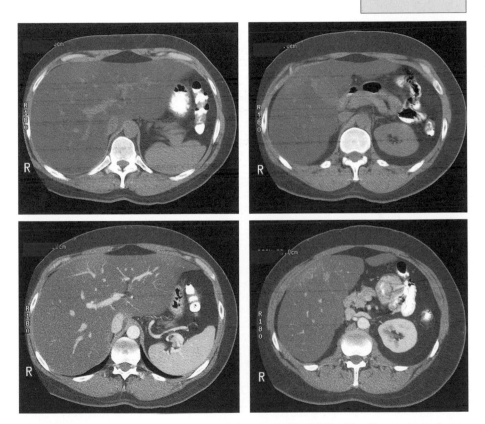

Sonographically suspected liver lesion in the medial segment of the left liver lobe. The unenhanced scans already show massive fatty degeneration of the liver with areas of less pronounced fatty degeneration, giving the liver a map-like appearance. Normal appearance of the vessels after i.v. administration of contrast material without signs of tumor.

Liver (search for hypovascularized metastases)

Region	entire liver
Scout view	256 mm, 120 kV, 50–100 mA, pa
Contrast media	i.v.: 120 ml non-ionic CM, iodine content: 300–320 mg/ml oral: 1000 ml over 60 min
Injection rate	2.5 ml/sec
Scan delay time	60 sec after start of bolus (portal venous phase)
CT technique	120 kV, 165–290 mA, 512 matrix, inspiration spiral: 24–32 rotations 8 mm slice thickness / 8 mm table feed (pitch 1:1) bottom to top
Reconstruction	4 mm interval, standard algorithm
Photography	12 on 1, patient information, scout view without and with cut lines, soft-tissue window from top to bottom, basal lung segments at lung window
Remarks	1. Have the patient drink a cup of water immediately before scanning for better filling of the stomach. 2. The reconstruction interval is 4 mm. To keep the number of images to be interpreted within reasonable limits, only alternate images should be photographed (corresponding to a reconstruction interval of 8 mm). In all unclear cases or if a CT scanner with a cine mode is available, the liver can be "leafed through" at the console. 3. Instruct the patient to breathe deeply before scanning. 4. If post-processing in 2D (multiplanar)/3D is required, the reconstruction interval should be 3 mm (approx. 30% of the nominal slice thickness). 5. The table feed can be increased up to 16 mm (pitch 2:1). 6. Obtain delayed scans after 5–10 min in patients with suspected cholangiocarcinoma or gallbladder carcinoma, since these tumors show a characteristic enhancement pattern in the late phase. 7. For oral CM administration, see "General remarks", page IX.

Brief protocol
CM oral, i.v. 120 ml 2.5 ml/sec 60 sec 8/8/4 bottom to top

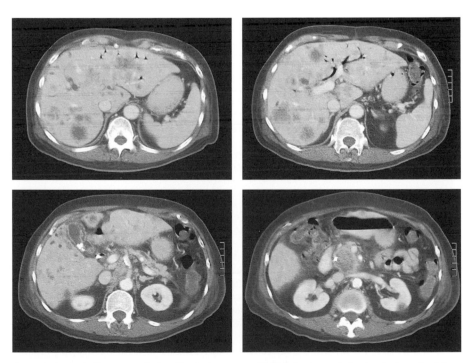

3-cm carcinoma in the pancreatic head/uncinate process. Multiple hypovascularized metastases in all liver segments, dilatation of the intrahepatic bile ducts, air in the bile ducts after ERCP, and placement of a stent in the common bile duct. Early retroperitoneal carcinomatosis with tumorous encasement of the celiac trunk. Maximal enhancement of hepatic parenchyma in the portal venous phase with optimal delineation of the hypovascularized liver lesions.

Liver (lesion characterization)

Region	liver lesion
Scout view	256 mm, 120 kV, 50–100 mA, pa
Unenhanced	120 kV, 110 mA, inspiration
	spiral: 12–24 rotations 8 mm slice thickness / 10 mm table feed (pitch 1.25:1) top to bottom scanning through the expected liver lesion
Contrast media	i.v.: 120 ml non-ionic CM, iodine content: 300–320 mg/ml no oral contrast material
Injection rate	4 ml/sec
Scan delay time	15 sec after start of bolus (arterial phase)
CT technique	120 kV, 65–210 mA, 512 matrix, inspiration, localize largest extension of lesion, followed by serial dynamic study
	dynamic: 10 mm slice thickness / 0 mm table feed 8 acquisitions every 3 sec, followed by 5 acquisitions every 10 sec, and 1 acquisition each after 2, 3, 4, and 5 min instruct patient to breathe after the initial 8 acquisitions, after the following 3, and then before each of the acquisitions at 1 min intervals
Reconstruction	standard algorithm
Photography	12 on 1, patient information, scout view without and with cut lines, soft-tissue window
Remarks	1. The dynamic CM enhanced study starting in the early arterial phase yields information for lesion characterization (in particular differentiation of FNH, adenoma, HCC, hemangioma). The patient has to be instructed prior to the examination to attain a similar degree of inspiration with each breath-hold for image acquisition at identical locations. 2. The dynamic study can be evaluated by means of an ROI (region of interest) placed in the lesion and plotting of a time/density curve. 3. The tube current should not exceed 210 mA per scan to minimize radiation exposure. 4. Giant lesions may require delayed scanning after 10 min.

**unenhanced
CM i.v.
120 ml
4 ml/sec
15 sec
dynamic series**

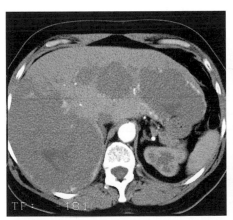 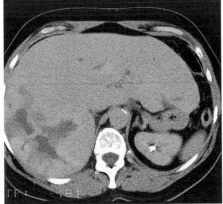

Serial scans at identical locations show lacuna-like contrast material pools in the periphery of the lesions during the early arterial phase. In the further course, there is fill-in and isointensity of the tumor with gaps corresponding to central, thrombotic areas in the late phase – typical dynamic enhancement pattern of giant hemangiomas.

CT during arterial portography (CTAP)

Region	entire liver
Scout view	256 mm, 120 kV, 50–100 mA, pa
Unenhanced	120 kV, 110–165 mA, inspiration
	spiral: 24–32 rotations 10 mm slice thickness / 10 mm table feed (pitch 1:1) top to bottom scanning through the upper abdomen
Contrast media	i.a.: 60 ml non-ionic CM, iodine content: 300–320 mg/ml, mixed 1:1 with 60 ml NaCl solution (total volume: 120 ml) injection via intra-arterial catheter with tip in the superior mesenteric artery or splenic artery
Injection rate	2 ml/sec
Scan delay time	40 sec after start of bolus
CT technique	120 kV, 220–290 mA, 512 matrix, inspiration
	spiral: 24–32 rotations 8 mm slice thickness / 8 mm table feed (pitch 1:1) bottom to top
Reconstruction	4 mm interval, soft-tissue algorithm
Photography	12 on 1, patient information, scout view without and with cut lines, unenhanced series and both CM enhanced series at soft-tissue window from top to bottom, basal lung segments at lung window (with edge enhancement if necessary)
Remarks	1. CTAP is at present the most sensitive modality for pre-operative detection of liver lesions, but it is not suitable for lesion characterization (see liver protocol for lesion characterization, page 80). 2. If post-processing in 2D (multiplanar)/3D is required, the reconstruction interval should be 3 mm (approx. 30% of the nominal slice thickness). 3. The pitch can be increased to 2:1.

unenhanced
CM i.a.
60/60 ml
(CM/NaCl)
2 ml/sec
40 sec
8/8/4
bottom to top

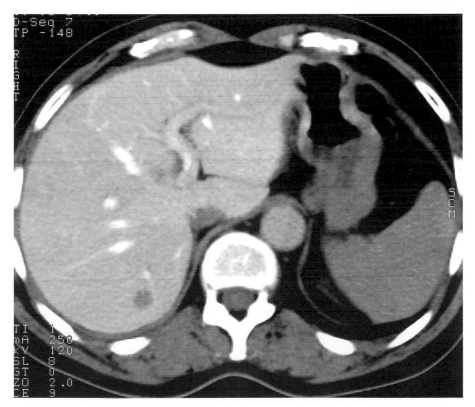

Following injection of contrast material via catheter in the superior mesenteric artery, there is portal opacification of the liver with delineation of a hypodense lesion in the 7th liver segment.

Pancreas (pancreatitis, follow-up)

Region	above diaphragm to below uncinate process
Scout view	256 mm, 120 kV, 50–100 mA, pa
Unenhanced	120 kV, 165 mA, inspiration
	spiral: 12–24 rotations 5 mm slice thickness / 10 mm table feed (pitch 2:1) top to bottom scanning through the upper abdomen
Contrast media	i.v.: 100 ml non-ionic CM, iodine content: 300–320 mg/ml oral: 500 ml over 15 min (only if clinically justifiable), the last cup immediately before scanning
Injection rate	2.5 ml/sec
Scan delay time	40 sec after start of bolus
CT technique	120 kV, 210–290 mA, 512 matrix, inspiration
	spiral: 12–24 rotations 5 mm slice thickness / 5 mm table feed (pitch 1:1) bottom to top scanning through the pancreas region, followed by
	incremental: dynamic screening 8 mm slice thickness / 8 mm table feed remainder of the liver to diaphragm, breaks for breathing
Reconstruction	10 mm interval for unenhanced scan, standard algorithm 5 mm interval for CM enhanced spiral, standard algorithm
Photography	12 on 1, patient information, scout view without and with cut lines, unenhanced scan at soft-tissue window from top to bottom, CM enhanced series at soft-tissue window from top to bottom, basal lung segments at lung window
Remarks	1. Normal tap water or carbonated mineral water can be used as an alternative to positive (radiodense) oral contrast material. This will make the duodenal wall appear bright (CM enhancement) against the lumen. Administer oral CM only if clinically justifiable . 2. Instruct the patient to breathe deeply before scanning. 3. If post-processing in 2D (multiplanar)/3D is required, the reconstruction interval should be 2 mm (approx. 30% of the nominal slice thickness). Use 3D protocol for assessment of vessel infiltration.

Brief protocol
unenhanced
CM oral, i.v.
100 ml
2.5 ml/sec
40 sec
5/5/5, 8/8
bottom to top

4. The table feed of the CM enhanced spiral can be increased up to 10 mm (pitch 2:1).
5. Enhancement as an expression of normal parenchymal perfusion can be quantified by comparing the pre- and post-contrast CT values in an ROI (region of interest) (typical values: post-contrast increase > 30 HU).
6. 1–2 single scans through the pelvis may be necessary, since severe forms of pancreatitis may be associated with free fluid accumulations in the pelvis.
7. For oral CM administration, see "General remarks", page IX.

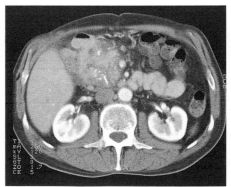 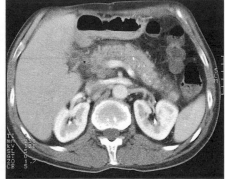

Acute episode of chronic calcifying pancreatitis. Stranding in peripancreatic fatty tissue in the area of the body and tail, slight exudation at the pancreatic head. Sufficient parenchymal opacification without demonstration of necrotic areas.

Pancreas (tumor search, tumor staging, 3D reconstruction)

Region	above diaphragm to below uncinate process
Scout view	256 mm, 120 kV, 50–100 mA, pa
Unenhanced	120 kV, 165 mA, inspiration
	spiral: 12–24 rotations 5 mm slice thickness / 10 mm table feed (pitch 2:1) top to bottom scanning through anticipated pancreatic region
Contrast media	i.v.: 140 ml non-ionic CM, iodine content: 300–320 mg/ml oral: 500 ml over 15 min, the last cup immediately before scanning
Injection rate	4 ml/sec
Scan delay time	60 sec after start of bolus
CT technique	120 kV, 210–290 mA, 512 matrix, inspiration
	spiral: 12–24 rotations 5 mm slice thickness / 5 mm table feed (pitch 1:1) bottom to top scanning through the pancreatic region, followed by
	incremental: dynamic screening 8 mm slice thickness / 8 mm table feed remainder of the liver to diaphragm, breaks for breathing
Reconstruction	10 mm interval for unenhanced scan, standard algorithm 3 mm interval for CM enhanced spiral, standard algorithm
Photography	12 on 1, patient information, scout view without and with cut lines, unenhanced scan at soft-tissue window from top to bottom, CM enhanced series at soft-tissue window from top to bottom, basal lung segments at lung window
Remarks	1. Normal tap water or carbonated mineral water can be used as an alternative to positive (radiodense) oral contrast material. This will make the duodenal wall appear bright (CM enhancement) against the lumen. Administer oral CM only if clinically justifiable. 2. Instruct the patient to breathe deeply before scanning. 4. For post-processing in 2D (multiplanar)/3D, the reconstruction interval of the pancreas spiral should be 2 mm (approx. 30% of the nominal slice thickness).

Brief protocol

5. The table feed of the CM enhanced spiral can be increased up to 10 mm (pitch 2:1).
6. In selected cases, it might be advantageous to inject 10–20 mg Glucagon® intravenously for optimal duodenal distension.
7. For oral CM administration, see "General remarks", page IX.

unenhanced
CM oral, i.v.
140 ml
4 ml/sec
60 sec
5/5/3
bottom to top

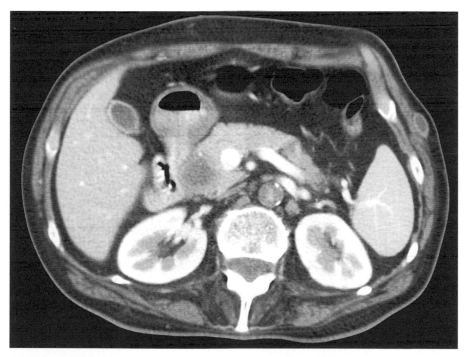

1.5-cm metastasis from bronchogenic carcinoma in the pancreatic head with compression of the duodenum opacified by oral contrast material. The hypodense lesion is clearly demarcated against the contrast-enhanced parenchyma. Accessory finding: occlusion of a subcutaneous bypass in Leriche's syndrome.

Kidneys

Region	kidneys
Scout view	256 mm, 120 kV, 50–100 mA, pa
Unenhanced	120 kV, 110 mA, inspiration
	spiral: 24 rotations
	8 mm slice thickness / 10 mm table feed (pitch 1.25:1)
	top to bottom scanning through anticipated kidney region
Contrast media	i.v.: 80 ml non-ionic CM, iodine content: 300–320 mg/ml
	oral: 1000 ml over 60 min
Injection rate	2 ml/sec
Scan delay time	40 sec after start of bolus
CT technique	120 kV, 110–290 mA, 512 matrix, inspiration
	spiral: 24 rotations
	5 mm slice thickness / 5 mm table feed (pitch 1:1)
	bottom to top
Reconstruction	5 mm interval, standard algorithm
Photography	12 on 1, patient information, scout view without and with cut lines, unenhanced and CM enhanced series at soft-tissue window from top to bottom

Remarks

1. For assessment of suspected thrombosis of the renal vein or inferior vena cava in patients with known malignancy, the scan delay should be 70 sec and the scanning area should extend to the right atrium.
2. For suspected renal artery stenosis, use the CT angiography protocol for renal arteries without oral administration of contrast material.
3. Instruct the patient to breathe deeply before scanning.
4. Sagittal 2D reconstruction with a reconstruction interval of 2 mm (approx. 30% of the nominal slice thickness) is recommended for evaluation of tumor extension.
5. The table feed can be increased up to 10 mm (pitch 2:1).
6. In case of a pathologic finding in the renal pelvis/ureter, delayed scanning with 100–150 mA after 5 min may be necessary. Alternatively, 20 ml contrast material for opacification of the renal pelvis/ureter may be administered about 5 min before scanning.

Brief protocol
unenhanced
CM oral, i.v.
80 ml
2 ml/sec
40 sec
5/5/5
bottom to top

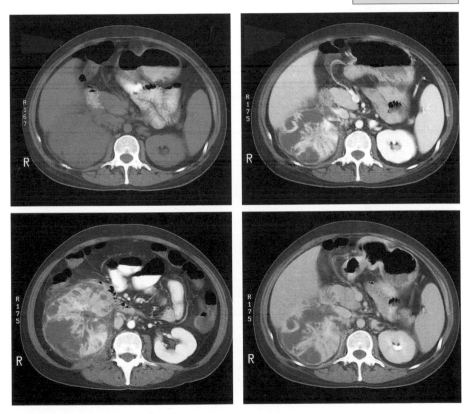

Xanthogranulomatous pyelonephritis. Scans before and after bolus administration of contrast material and delayed scanning after 5 minutes.

Adrenals glands

Region	adrenals
Scout view	256 mm, 120 kV, 50–100 mA, pa
Unenhanced	120 kV, 65–165 mA, inspiration
	spiral: 24 rotations 5 mm slice thickness / 5 mm table feed (pitch 1:1) top to bottom scanning through expected adrenal region
Contrast media	i.v.: 120 ml non-ionic CM, iodine content: 300–320 mg/ml
Injection rate	2.5 ml/sec
Scan delay time	50 sec after start of bolus
CT technique	120 kV, 65–210 mA, inspiration
	spiral: 12–24 rotations 5 mm slice thickness / 5 mm table feed (pitch 1:1) top to bottom, only adrenals as determined on the unenhanced images
Reconstruction	3 mm interval for pre-contrast scans and for CM enhanced series if required, standard algorithm, magnified reconstruction of scans containing adrenals (smaller FOV)
Photography	12 on 1, patient information, scout view without and with cut lines, unenhanced series, magnification, CM enhanced series if applicable, soft-tissue window from top to bottom

Only for adrenal tumors (diameter > 2.5 cm)

Remarks	1. The risk of inducing a hypertensive crisis in patients with pheochromocytoma by intravenous administration of contrast material is discussed controversially in the literature. We recommend that phentolamine for intravenous injection (Regitin®) should be readily available for emergencies.. 2. In patients with clinically suspected pheochromocytoma and no adrenal abnormalities, scanning should be extended to the area of the aortic bifurcation and, if necessary, to the urinary bladder after CM administration to exclude extra-adrenal localization (Zuckerkandl's organ). 3. The tube current should not exceed 75 mA in slender patients.

Brief protocol
unenhanced
CM i.v.
if required
120 ml
2.5 ml/sec
50 sec
5/5/3
top to bottom

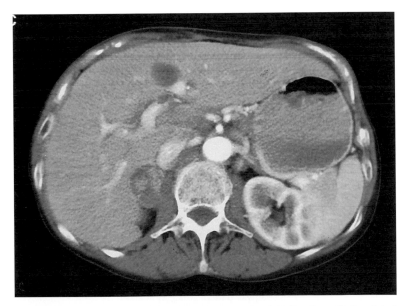

Heterogeneous enhancement of the adrenal mass on the right. Together with the clinical presentation, this enhancement pattern is indicative of pheochromocytoma.

Paranasal sinuses

Region	posterior wall of sphenoidal sinuses to anterior wall of frontal sinuses
Scout view	256 mm, 120 kV, 50 mA, lateral
Contrast media	–
Injection rate	–
Scan delay time	–
CT technique	120 kV, 65–165 mA, 512 matrix
	patient in prone position with reclined head, gantry inclination perpendicular to orbital floor (coronal section)
	spiral: 12 rotations 5 mm slice thickness / 10 mm table feed (pitch 2:1) posterior to anterior
Reconstruction	5 mm interval, lung/bone algorithm
Photography	12 on 1, patient information, scout view without and with cut lines, soft-tissue window from posterior to anterior, bone window from posterior to anterior
Remarks	1. Since the lenses are in the scanning area, strict indication and minimal tube current ($\leq$ 65 mA) are mandatory. A pitch of 2:1 further reduces the x-ray dose by a factor of 2.
	2. Use a 2 mm interval for multiplanar reconstruction of the data set in the axial direction.
	3. Multiple radiodense tooth fillings may produce artifacts in coronal sections and considerably impair interpretation. Such artifacts can be avoided by axial scanning with coronal reconstruction.
	4. For highly detailed resolution, we recommend a scan time of 2 sec and conventional, incremental scanning at a slice thickness of 5 mm.
	5. For pre-operative planning, the reconstruction interval in the area of the anterior ethmoidal cells (orifices!) may have to be changed to 3 mm.
	6. For tumor staging, an axial examination of the frontal skull and neck is recommended after 120 ml of i.v. CM, injection rate 2 ml/sec, 70 sec scan delay, 5/5/5, as well as coronal reconstruction in the area of the paranasal sinuses (with a reconstruction interval of 2 mm).

Brief protocol

**unenhanced
5/10/5
coronal
low-dose
technique**

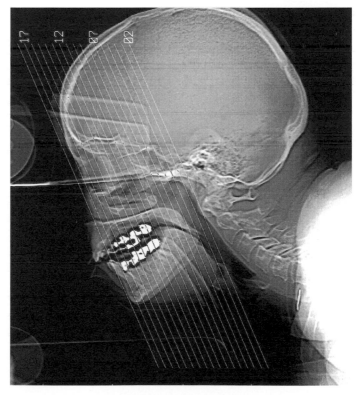

Lateral scout view. Patient in prone position with reclined head. A precise coronal slice orientation can typically be achieved with a gantry inclination of 10–25˚.

Dental CT (with multiplanar reconstruction)

Region	entire maxilla or mandible, depending on diagnostic problem
Scout view	256 mm, 120 kV, 50 mA, lateral
Contrast media	–
Injection rate	–
Scan delay time	–
CT technique	120 kV, 65 mA, 512 matrix, 2 sec scan time
	patient in supine position with fixed head, gantry inclination parallel to the branch of jaw to be examined, place cellulose or a non-radiodense wedge between the teeth
	no spiral, 1.5 mm slice thickness / 1 mm table feed
Reconstruction	lung/bone algorithm
Postprocessing	multiplanar sectioning along the row of teeth, coronal (image similar to OPTG) and sagittal (perpendicular to the branch of jaw)
Photography	patient information, scout view, 12 on 1 for coronal sections, 36 on 1 for sagittal sections, bone window
Remarks	1. The slice thickness should not be greater than 2 mm since partial volume effects may reduce the delineation of the mandibular canal and other structures. 2. The energy per section should not exceed 130 mA. 3. Securely fix the patient's head.

Brief protocol

unenhanced
1.5/1
axial, 65 mA
multiplanar
reconstruction
coronal/sagittal

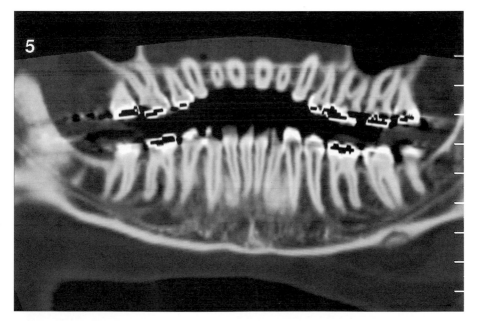

Osteomyelitis with development of a small bone sequestrum at the left mandible. The alveolar canal is not involved in the process.

CT angiography:
Thoracic aortic aneurysm (TAA)

Region	above clavicles to below diaphragm
Scout view	450 mm, 120 kV, 50–100 mA, pa
Contrast media	i.v.: 90 ml non-ionic CM, iodine content: 300–320 mg/ml
Injection rate	3 ml/sec
Scan delay time	20 sec after start of bolus
CT technique	120 kV, 110–220 mA, 512 matrix, inspiration spiral: 24–32 rotations 5 mm slice thickness / 8 mm table feed (pitch 1.6:1) top to bottom
Reconstruction	5 mm interval, standard algorithm
Postprocessing	multiplanar sectioning along the aorta, coronal and sagittal reconstructions, MIP or surface rendering
Photography	12 on 1, patient information, scout view without and with cut lines, axial sections (every 2nd section) at soft-tissue window, reconstructions (multiplanar, MIP, surface) in pertinent projections
Remarks	1. Use a reconstruction interval of 2 mm for post-processing. 2. Depending on the surgical problem, visualization of the thoracic origins (intercostal arteries) may be important and requires selective reconstruction of the aorta from the raw data. 3. Multiplanar reconstruction along a path does not require additional editing. Display several sections parallel to the path. Distance measurements represent true distances. 4. MIP requires editing, e.g. removal of the vertebral column and ribs. This may be done section per section or along a path on the sagittal image. Separation of aortic calcifications may be difficult. 5. 3D surface displays may be generated by editing or by establishment of a threshold value. Best pre-operative procedure for 3D display. 6. Instruct the patient to breathe deeply before scanning and point out that smooth breathing is allowed in case of shortness of breath.

Brief protocol
CM i.v. 90 ml 3 ml/sec 20 sec 5/8/5 top to bottom

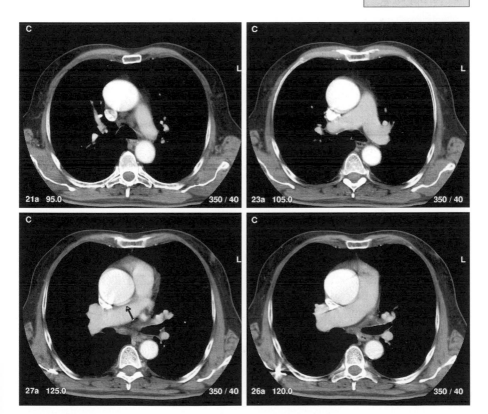

Dilatation of the ascending aorta in a patient with aortic valve stenosis without signs of dissection. The double contour (arrow) of the ascending aorta is caused by pulsation.

CT angiography:
Abdominal aortic aneurysm (AAA)

Region	above diaphragm to level of hip joints
Scout view	512 mm, 120 kV, 50–100 mA, pa
Contrast media	i.v.: 100 ml non-ionic CM, iodine content: 300–320 mg/ml
Injection rate	3 ml/sec
Scan delay time	20 sec after start of bolus
CT technique	120 kV, 165–220 mA, 512 matrix, inspiration
	spiral: 24–32 rotations 5 mm slice thickness / 10 mm table feed (pitch 2:1) top to bottom
Reconstruction	5 mm interval, standard algorithm
Postprocessing	multiplanar sectioning along the aorta, coronal and sagittal reconstructions, MIP or surface rendering
Photography	12 on 1, patient information, scout view without and with cut lines, axial sections (every 2nd section at soft-tissue window, reconstructions (multiplanar, MIP, surface) in pertinent projections
Remarks	1. Use a reconstruction interval of 3 mm for post-processing. 2. Multiplanar reconstruction along a path does not require additional editing. Display several sections parallel to the path. Distance measurements represent true distances. 3. MIP requires editing, e.g. removal of the vertebral column. This may be done section per section or along a path on the sagittal image. Separation of aortic calcifications may be difficult. 4. 3D surface displays may be generated by editing or by establishment of a threshold value. Best pre-operative procedure for 3D display. 5. Instruct the patient to breathe deeply before scanning and point out that smooth breathing is allowed in case of shortness of breath. 6. Do not give oral contrast material (impairs identification of vessels on 3D images).

Brief protocol

CM i.v.
100 ml
3 ml/sec
20 sec
5/10/5
top to bottom

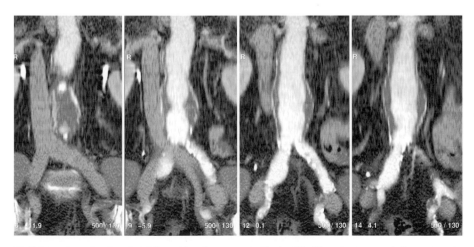

Multiplanar reconstruction of an infrarenal aortic aneurysm. The length of the aneurysm made it necessary to increase the beam collimation to 8 mm with a table feed of 16 mm/sec.

CT angiography:
Thoracic and abdominal aortic aneurysm

Region	above clavicles to level of hip joints
Scout view	512 mm, 120 kV, 50–100 mA, pa
Contrast media	i.v.: 90 ml (chest) + 70 ml (abdomen) non-ionic CM, iodine content: 300–320 mg/ml
Injection rate	2.5 ml/sec
Scan delay time	20 sec after start of bolus
CT technique	120 kV, 110–290 mA, 512 matrix, inspiration
	1st spiral: chest 24–32 rotations 5 mm slice thickness / 10 mm table feed (pitch 2:1) top to bottom
	start second bolus
	2nd spiral: abdomen 5 mm slice thickness / 10 mm table feed (pitch 2:1) top to bottom
Reconstruction	5 mm interval, standard algorithm
Postprocessing	multiplanar sectioning along the aorta, coronal and sagittal reconstructions, MIP or surface rendering
Photography	12 on 1, patient information, scout view without and with cut lines, axial sections (every 2nd section) at soft-tissue window, reconstructions (multiplanar, MIP, surface) in pertinent projections
Remarks	1. Shallow breathing negligibly affects image quality in the pelvic area. 2. Use a reconstruction interval of 3 mm for post-processing. 3. For assessing the extent of dissection and involvement of aortic branches such as cranial vessels, renal arteries or mesenteric arteries, these areas should be scanned with a 3rd spiral at a slice thickness of 3 mm and a variable pitch (1:1 to 2:1) during breath-hold. Give second contrast bolus of 60 ml, 2 ml/sec, scan delay 25 sec; reconstruction interval of 1 mm for multiplanar reconstruction.

Brief protocol
CM i.v. **90/70 ml** **2.5 ml/sec** **20 sec** **5/10/5** **top to bottom**

4. Multiplanar reconstruction along a path does not require additional editing. Display several sections parallel to the path. Distance measurements represent true distances.
5. MIP requires editing, e.g. removal of the vertebral column and ribs. This may be done section per section or along a path on the sagittal image. Separation of aortic calcifications may be difficult.
6. 3D surface displays may be generated by editing or by establishment of a threshold value. Best preoperative procedure for 3D display.
7. Instruct the patient to breathe deeply before scanning and point out that smooth breathing is allowed in case of shortness of breath.

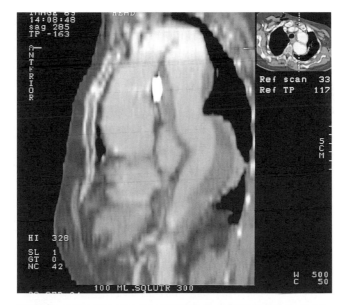

Sagittal reconstruction of a non-dissecting thoraco-abdominal aneurysm. Endobronchial stent because of compression of the left primary bronchus between the ectatic ascending and descending aorta.

CT angiography:
Renal arteries

Region	renal arteries
Scout view	256 mm, 120 kV, 50–100 mA, pa
Unenhanced	120 kV, 65–110 mA, inspiration spiral: 12 rotations 10 mm slice thickness / 10 mm table feed (pitch 1:1) top to bottom
Contrast media	i.v.: 90 ml non-ionic CM, iodine content: 300–320 mg/ml
Injection rate	3 ml/sec
Scan delay time	25 sec after start of bolus
CT technique	120 kV, 110–290 mA, 512 matrix, inspiration spiral: 24–32 rotations 2 mm slice thickness / 3 mm table feed (pitch 1.5:1) top to bottom, only area of the renal arteries as determined on the unenhanced image. The origin of the renal arteries should be in the upper third of the spiral (descending course of the arteries)
Reconstruction	1 mm interval, standard algorithm
Postprocessing	multiplanar sectioning along the renal arteries, coronal and axial reconstructions, MIP or surface rendering
Photography	12 on 1, patient information, scout view without and with cut lines, axial sections (every 3rd section at soft-tissue window, reconstructions (multiplanar, MIP, surface) in pertinent projections
Remarks	1. Multiplanar reconstruction along a path does not require additional editing. Display several sections parallel to the path. Distance measurements represent true distances. 2. MIP requires editing, e.g. removal of the vertebral column. This may be done section per section or along a path on the sagittal image. Separation of aortic calcifications may be difficult. 3. 3D surface displays may be generated by editing or by establishment of a threshold value. Note: the former bears the risk of misinterpretation of anatomical structures, the latter cannot differentiate partial volume effects from true density values which may lead to over- or underestimation of stenoses or even creation of pseudostenoses. 4. Instruct the patient to breathe deeply before scanning.

Brief protocol
CM i.v.
90 ml
3 ml/sec
25 sec
2/3/1
top to bottom

5. Reduction of the slice thickness to 1.5 or 1 mm will increase resolution along the z-axis. Most tubes have a maximal capacity of only 150 mA when a small focus is used, which increases image noise and thus impairs image quality. Soft filters compensate for noise at the expense of spatial resolution.

6. The table feed can be increased up to 4 mm (pitch 2:1).

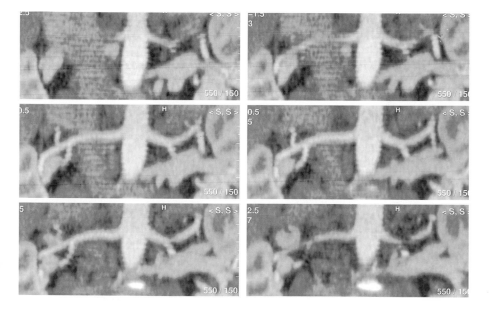

26-year-old female with hypertension. The coronal reconstruction shows a normal origin and course of the renal arteries without signs of stenosis.

Cardiac CT (with multiplanar reconstruction)

Region	aortic arch to apex of heart
Scout view	256 mm, 120 kV, 50–100 mA, lateral
Contrast media	i.v.: 60 ml non-ionic CM, iodine content: 300–320 mg/ml
Injection rate	2.5 ml/sec
Scan delay time	30 sec after start of bolus
CT technique	120 kV, 110–220 mA, 512 matrix, inspiration maximal gantry inclination parallel to the long heart axis spiral: 24–32 rotations 10 mm slice thickness / 10 mm table feed (pitch 1:1) bottom to top
Reconstruction	5 mm interval, standard algorithm (without post-processing) 3 mm interval, standard algorithm (for post-processing)
Postprocessing	multiplanar sectioning along the long heart axis every 3 mm, corresponding to a coronal heart section
Photography	12 on 1, patient information, scout view without and with cut lines, 5 mm original scans and reconstructions at soft-tissue window, original scans at lung window (with edge enhancement if necessary)
Remarks	1. To facilitate evaluation, axial sections can be calculated from the original data by multiplanar reconstruction. 2. Increase scan delay to 40 sec in patients with known heart failure. 3. Reduction of the table feed and slice thickness, e.g. 5/5/5, does not improve image quality, since image quality will be affected by more heart beats. Alternatively, a spiral with 5 mm slice thickness and 10 mm table feed can be used (pitch 2:1). 4. Instruct the patient to breathe deeply before scanning.

Brief protocol

CM i.v.
60 ml
2.5 ml/sec
30 sec
10/10/5
bottom to top

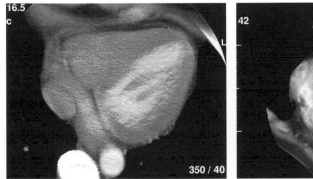
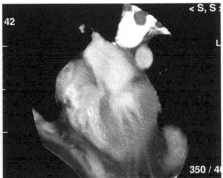

Continuous peripheral intravenous administration of contrast material with initial enhancement of the left ventricle only. A second spiral with multiplanar reconstruction along the long heart axis shows a patent oval foramen.

Incremental CT

Abdomen and pelvis

Region	above diaphragm to pubic symphysis
Scout view	512 mm, 120 kV, 50–100 mA, pa
Contrast media	i.v.: 140 ml non-ionic CM, iodine content: 300–320 mg/ml oral: 1000 ml over 60 min rectal: 500 ml immediately before scanning
Injection rate	2.5 ml/sec for 20 sec 1.5 ml/sec for 60 sec
Scan delay time	40 sec after start of bolus
CT technique	120 kV, 150–300 mA, 512 matrix, inspiration 8 mm slice thickness / 8 mm table feed top to bottom
Reconstruction	standard algorithm
Photography	12 on 1, patient information, scout view without and with cut lines, soft-tissue window, basal lung segments at lung window
Remarks	1. Have the patient drink a cup of water immediately before scanning for better filling of the stomach. 2. Instruct the patient to breathe deeply before scanning. 3. In case of a pathologic finding in the kidneys, ureters, or bladder, delayed scanning with 150–200 mA after 5 min may be necessary. 4. Rectal CM administration should be performed for all gynecological examinations and suspected pathology in the colon/rectum. As an alternative to a contrast enema, a pre-packaged implementation device (approx. 150 ml) can be used. 5. Co-administration of 20 mg metoclopramide (MCP) with the first cup of contrast material accelerates the CM passage. 6. For oral and rectal CM administration, see "General remarks", page IX.

Brief protocol
CM oral, rectal i.v.
140 ml
2.5/1.5 ml/sec
40 sec
8/8
top to bottom

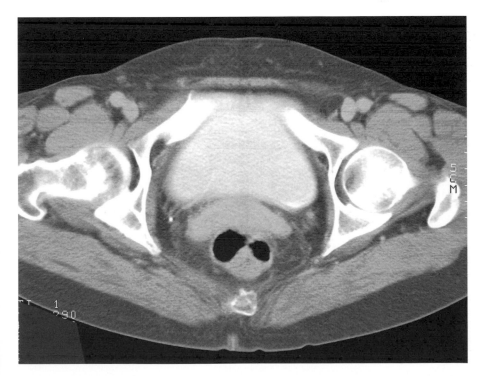

Rectal carcinoma, 2 cm in diameter, and local lymphadenopathy. Since the tumor was already palpable at the digital examination, rectal CM was not given because of the risk of perforation.

Chest and upper abdomen

Region	above clavicles to lower kidney pole
Scout view	512 mm, 120 kV, 50–100 mA, pa
Contrast media	i.v.: 120 ml (abdomen) + 40 ml (chest) non-ionic CM, iodine content: 300–320 mg/ml oral: 1000 ml over 60 min
Injection rate	2.5 ml/sec for 20 sec, 1.5 ml/sec for 45 sec (abdomen bolus) 1 ml/sec (chest bolus)
Scan delay time	40 sec after start of first bolus, 10 sec after start of second bolus
CT technique	120 kV, 100–300 mA, 512 matrix, inspiration 8 mm slice thickness / 8 mm table feed top to bottom, above diaphragm to lower kidney pole start chest bolus 8 mm slice thickness / 8 mm table feed top to bottom, above clavicles to diaphragm
Reconstruction	standard algorithm (abdomen) lung/bone algorithm (chest)
Photography	12 on 1, patient information, scout view without and with cut lines, soft-tissue window, lung window
Remarks	1. Have the patient drink a cup of water immediately before scanning for better filling of the stomach. 2. Instruct the patient to breathe deeply before scanning. 3. In case of a pathologic finding in the renal pelvis/ureter, delayed scanning after 5 min may be necessary. 4. For oral CM administration, see "General remarks", page IX.

Brief protocol

CM oral, i.v.
120/40 ml
2.5/1.5/1 ml/sec,
40/10 sec
8/8
top to bottom

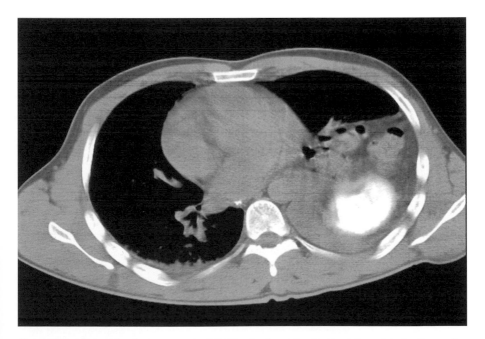

Status post rupture of the diaphragm on the left. Visualization of the displaced stomach in the thorax after repeated administration of oral contrast material.

Neck and chest

Region	below base of skull to below both sinuses of diaphragm include adrenals in bronchogenic carcinoma
Scout view	512 mm, 120 kV, 50–100 mA, pa
Contrast media	i.v.: 120 ml (chest) + 40 ml (neck) non-ionic CM, iodine content: 300–320 mg/ml
Injection rate	2 ml/sec for 30 sec, 1.5 ml/sec for 45 sec (chest scan) 1.5 ml/sec (neck scan)
Scan delay time	30 sec after start of chest bolus, 10 sec after start of neck bolus
CT technique	120 kV, 100–200 mA, inspiration 8 mm slice thickness / 8 mm table feed top to bottom, above clavicles to below both sinuses reposition patient with arms parallel to trunk, start neck bolus 5 mm slice thickness / 5 mm table feed top to bottom, below base of skull to above clavicles
Reconstruction	lung/bone algorithm (chest) standard algorithm (neck)
Photography	12 on 1, patient information, scout view without and with cut lines, soft-tissue window, lung window
Remarks	1. A suitable contrast agent for the esophagus is Esopho-Cat® (2 tablespoons immediately before scanning). 2. Edge enhancement (implemented in most scanners as a post-processing function) facilitates the detection of very small intrapulmonary nodules. 3. Follow-up of intrapulmonary nodules during therapy may be done without intravenous administration of contrast material. 4. The tube current should not exceed 100 mA in slender patients.

CM i.v.
120/40 ml
2/1.5 ml/sec
30/10 sec
8/8, 5/5
top to bottom

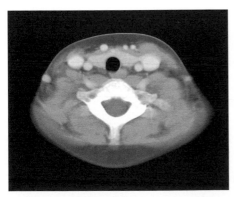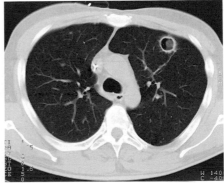

Indication: fever, questionable swelling of neck lymph nodes. Normal findings in the area of the neck. Reliable exclusion of enlarged lymph nodes by intravenous administration of contrast material. Demonstration of a typical aspergilloma in the left upper lobe of the lung.

Chest, abdomen, and pelvis

Region	above clavicles to pubic symphysis
Scout view	512 mm, 120 kV, 50–100 mA, pa
Contrast media	i.v.: 140 ml (abdomen and pelvis) + 40 ml (chest) non-ionic CM, iodine content: 300–320 mg/ml oral: 1000 ml over 60 min rectal: 500 ml immediately before scanning
Injection rate	2.5 ml/sec for 20 sec, 1.5 ml/sec for 60 sec (abdomen and pelvis) 1 ml/sec (chest bolus)
Scan delay time	40 sec after start of bolus, 10 sec after start of chest bolus
CT technique	120 kV, 100–300 mA, 512 matrix, inspiration 8 mm slice thickness / 8 mm table feed top to bottom, above diaphragm to symphysis start chest bolus 8 mm slice thickness / 8 mm table feed top to bottom, above clavicles to diaphragm
Reconstruction	standard algorithm (abdomen and pelvis) lung/bone algorithm (chest)
Photography	12 on 1, patient information, scout view without and with cut lines, soft-tissue window, lung window
Remarks	1. Have the patient drink a cup of water immediately before scanning for better filling of the stomach. 2. Instruct the patient to breathe deeply before scanning. 3. In case of a pathologic finding in the kidney, ureters, or bladder, delayed scanning after 5 min may be necessary. 4. Rectal CM administration should be performed for all gynecological examinations and suspected pathology in the colon/rectum. As an alternative to a contrast enema, a pre-packaged implementation device (approx. 150 ml) can be used. 5. Co-administration of 20 mg metoclopramide (MCP) with the first cup of contrast material accelerates the CM passage. 6. For oral and rectal CM administration, see "General remarks", page IX.

Brief protocol
CM oral, rectal
i.v.
140/40 ml
2.5/1.5/1 ml/sec
40/10 sec
8/8
top to bottom

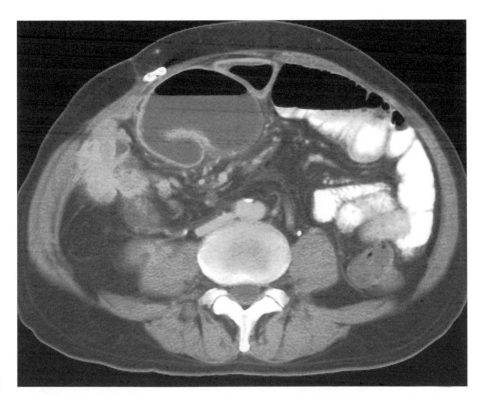

Recurrent colon carcinoma after hemicolectomy. Pronounced enhancement of the tumor and satisfactory opacification of the aorta. Opacification of the small intestine up to the stenosis (ileus) by the oral contrast material.

Neck, chest, abdomen, and pelvis

Region	below base of skull to pubic symphysis
Scout view	512 mm, 120 kV, 50–100 mA, pa, set upper limit to base of skull
Contrast media	i.v.: 140 ml (abdomen and pelvis) + 40 ml (chest) + 20 ml (neck) non-ionic CM, iodine content: 300–320 mg/ml oral: 1000 ml over 60 min rectal: 500 ml immediately before scanning
Injection rate	2.5 ml/sec for 20 sec, 1.5 ml/sec for 60 sec (abdomen and pelvis) 1 ml/sec (chest and neck bolus)
Scan delay time	40 sec after start of bolus, 10 sec after start of chest bolus 10 sec after start of neck bolus
CT technique	120 kV, 100–300 mA, 512 matrix, inspiration 8 mm slice thickness / 8 mm table feed top to bottom, above diaphragm to symphysis start chest bolus 8 mm slice thickness / 8 mm table feed top to bottom, above clavicles to diaphragm reposition patient's arms, start neck bolus 5 mm slice thickness / 5 mm table feed top to bottom, below base of skull to above clavicle
Reconstruction	standard algorithm (abdomen, pelvis, and neck) lung/bone algorithm (chest)
Photography	12 on 1, patient information, scout view without and with cut lines, soft-tissue window, lung window
Remarks	1. Since the chest and abdomen bolus may obscure neck pathology (tumors), we recommend to examine the neck or chest/neck separately from the abdomen/pelvis (at least 6 hours apart). 2. Have the patient drink a cup of water immediately before scanning for better filling of the stomach. 3. Instruct the patient to breathe deeply before scanning. 4. In case of a pathologic finding in the kidneys, ureters, or bladder, delayed scanning after 5 min may be necessary.

Brief protocol

5. Co-administration of 20 mg metoclopramide (MCP) with the first cup of contrast material accelerates the CM passage.
6. Rectal CM administration should be performed for all gynecological examinations and suspected pathology in the colon/rectum. As an alternative to a contrast enema, a pre-packaged implementation device (approx. 150 ml) can be used.
7. For oral and rectal CM administration, see "General remarks", page IX.

CM oral, rectal
i.v.
140/40/20 ml
2.5/1.5/1 ml/sec
40/10/10 sec
8/8, 5/5
top to bottom

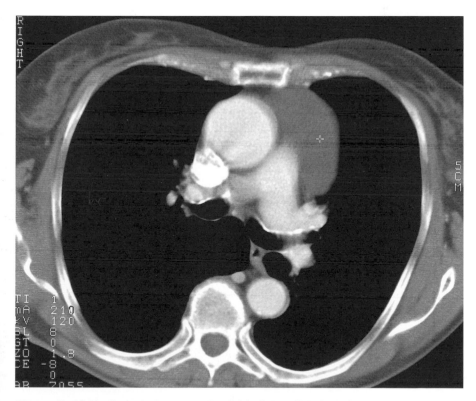

Circumscribed fluid collection in the upper pericardial duplicature. Vortexing in the superior vena cava with moderate artifact formation during influx of contrast material.

Neck

Region	below base of skull to tip of lung or to above aortic arch if required
Scout view	256 mm, 120 kV, 50–100 mA, lateral
Contrast media	i.v.: 80 ml non-ionic CM, iodine content: 300–320 mg/ml
Injection rate	2 ml/sec
Scan delay time	30 sec after start of bolus
CT technique	120 kV, 50–150 mA, inspiration incline gantry parallel to intervertebral disc C4–C5 5 mm slice thickness / 5 mm table feed top to bottom
Reconstruction	standard algorithm
Photography	12 on 1, patient information, scout view without and with cut lines, soft-tissue window, scans containing lung segments at lung window
Remarks	1. For the assessment of tumor extension (but not for lymph node staging), the scan delay may be increased to 60 sec and the amount of CM should be 120 ml. 2. Ask the patient not to swallow during scans. 3. The tube current should not be greater than 50 mA in patients with a slender neck.

Brief protocol
CM i.v. **80 ml** **2 ml/sec** **30 sec** **5/5** **top to bottom**

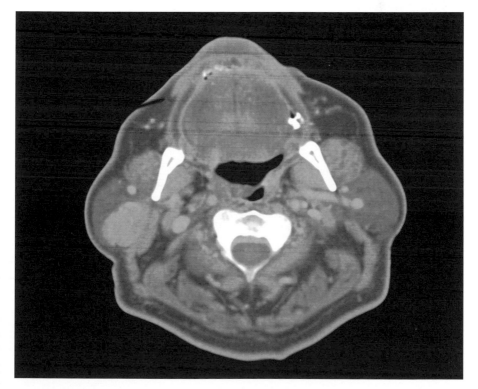

Pleomorphic adenoma of the right parotid gland. Weak opacification of the arteries and veins and pronounced tumor enhancement.

Chest

Region	above clavicles to below both sinuses of diaphragm include adrenals in bronchogenic carcinoma
Scout view	256 mm, 120 kV, 50–100 mA, pa
Contrast media	i.v.: 140 ml non-ionic CM, iodine content: 300–320 mg/ml
Injection rate	2 ml/sec for 30 sec 1 ml/sec for 60 sec
Scan delay time	15 sec after start of bolus
CT technique	120 kV, 100–200 mA, inspiration 8 mm slice thickness / 8 mm table feed top to bottom, extend scanning area to below both adrenals if required
Reconstruction	lung/bone algorithm
Photography	12 on 1, patient information, scout view without and with cut lines, soft-tissue window, lung window (with additional edge enhancement if required)
Remarks	1. A suitable contrast agent for the esophagus is Esopho-Cat® (2 tablespoons immediately before scanning). 2. Edge enhancement (implemented in most scanners as a post-processing function) facilitates the detection of very small lung lesions. 3. Follow-up of intrapulmonary nodules during therapy may be done without intravenous administration of contrast material. 4. The tube current should be reduced to a minimum in slender patients.

Brief protocol
CM i.v.
140 ml
2/1 ml/sec
15 sec
8/8
top to bottom

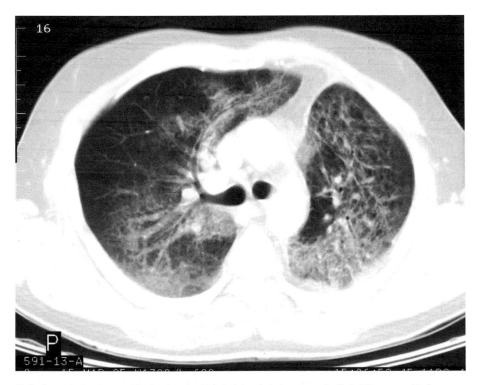

Reticular and alveolar opacification in mixed bacterial and viral pneumonia. Both hili appeared to be unremarkable.

Chest in HR technique (high-resolution technique)

Region	tip of lung to below both sinuses of diaphragm
Scout view	256 mm, 120 kV, 50–100 mA, pa
Contrast media	–
Injection rate	–
Scan delay time	–
CT technique	137 kV, 100–200 mA, 512 matrix, 1–2 sec scan time, inspiration
	1–2 mm slice thickness / 10 mm table feed top to bottom, allow patient to breathe after 3–5 scans (≈20 sec)
Reconstruction	lung/bone algorithm
Photography	12 on 1, patient information, scout view without and with cut lines, soft-tissue window, lung window
Remarks	1. This protocol can only be used for assessing interstitial pulmonary changes or bronchiectasis. The 8–9 mm interscan gap limits the assessment of mediastinal lymphadenopathy or intrapulmonary nodules.
	2. If contrast-enhanced scans are required, use chest protocol (see page 120).
	3. If subpleurally increased interstitial reticulation (basal/dorsal) is noted, turn patient to prone position and acquire single scans through this area after 5 min (thereby excluding purely orthostatic changes).
	4. With a scan time of 2 sec per section, more raw data can be acquired than with 1-sec scans, which improves contrast and resolution of details.
	5. The tube current should not exceed 100 mA in slender patients.

Brief protocol

**unenhanced
1–2/10
top to bottom**

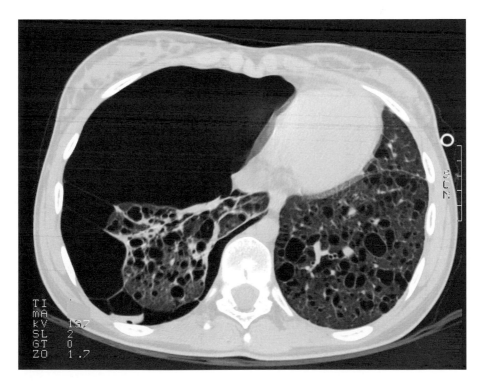

Idiopathic pulmonary fibrosis with rupture of a bulla and development of a valvular pneumothorax.

Upper abdomen

Region	above diaphragm to lower kidney pole
Scout view	256 mm, 120 kV, 50–100 mA, pa
Contrast media	i.v.: 140 ml non-ionic CM, iodine content: 300–320 mg/ml oral: 1000 ml over 60 min
Injection rate	2.5 ml/sec for 20 sec 1.5 ml/sec for 60 sec
Scan delay time	40 sec after start of bolus
CT technique	120 kV, 150–300 mA, 512 matrix, inspiration 8 mm slice thickness / 8 mm table feed top to bottom
Reconstruction	standard algorithm
Photography	12 on 1, patient information, scout view without and with cut lines, soft-tissue window, basal lung segments at lung window
Remarks	1. Have the patient drink a cup of water immediately before scanning for better filling of the stomach. 2. Instruct the patient to breathe deeply before scanning. 3. In case of a pathologic finding in the renal pelvis/ureter, delayed scanning after 5 min may be necessary. 4. For oral CM administration, see "General remarks", page IX.

Brief protocol

CM oral, i.v.
140 ml
2.5/1.5 ml/sec
40 sec
8/8
top to bottom

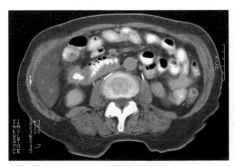 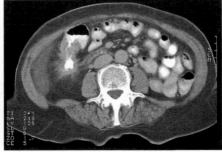

Colon carcinoma in the area of the right flexure with extensive infiltration of surrounding tissue and opacified residual lumen.

Pelvis

Region	lower kidney pole to pubic symphysis
Scout view	256 mm, 120 kV, 50–100 mA, pa
Contrast media	i.v.: 140 ml non-ionic CM, iodine content: 300–320 mg/ml oral: 1000 ml over 60 min rectal: 500 ml immediately before scanning
Injection rate	2.5 ml/sec
Scan delay time	50 sec after start of bolus
CT technique	120 kV, 150–300 mA, 512 matrix, inspiration 8 mm slice thickness / 8 mm table feed top to bottom
Reconstruction	standard algorithm
Photography	12 on 1, patient information, scout view without and with cut lines, soft-tissue window
Remarks	1. Beam-hardening artifacts at the level of the hip joints when the bladder is filled with contrast material make it very difficult to assess the pelvic wall in suspected lymphadenopathy. 2. Acquire delayed scans with CM filled bladder only for assessment of bladder pathology. 3. Minimize energy (≤150 mAs) especially in younger patients! 4. Always administer contrast material rectally. As an alternative to a contrast enema, a pre-packaged implementation device (approx. 150 ml) can be used. 5. Co-administration of 20 mg metoclopramide (MCP) with the first cup of contrast material accelerates the CM passage. 6. For oral and rectal CM administration, see "General remarks", page IX.

Brief protocol
CM oral, rectal i.v. 140 ml 2.5 ml/sec 50 sec 8/8 top to bottom

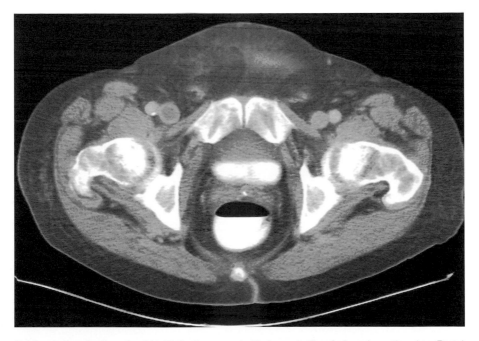

Pelvic vein thrombosis on the right. Wall enhancement with demonstration of a hypodense thrombus. Rectal administration of water-soluble contrast material.

Liver

Region	entire liver
Scout view	256 mm, 120 kV, 50–100 mA, pa
Contrast media	i.v.: 120 ml non-ionic CM, iodine content: 300–320 mg/ml oral: 1000 ml over 60 min
Injection rate	2.5 ml/sec for 20 sec 1.5 ml/sec for 45 sec
Scan delay time	40 sec after start of bolus
CT technique	120 kV, 150–300 mA, 512 matrix, inspiration 8 mm slice thickness / 8 mm table feed top to bottom
Reconstruction	standard algorithm
Photography	12 on 1, patient information, scout view without and with cut lines, soft-tissue window, basal lung segments at lung window
Remarks	1. In case of suspected hypervascularized metastases such as metastases from renal cell carcinoma, melanoma, breast cancer, or endocrine tumors, the CM enhanced series should be preceded by unenhanced scanning. Parameters: 8 mm slice thickness and 8 mm table feed. 2. For oral CM administration, see "General remarks", page IX.

Brief protocol

CM oral, i.v.
120 ml
2.5/1.5 ml/sec
40 sec
8/8
top to bottom

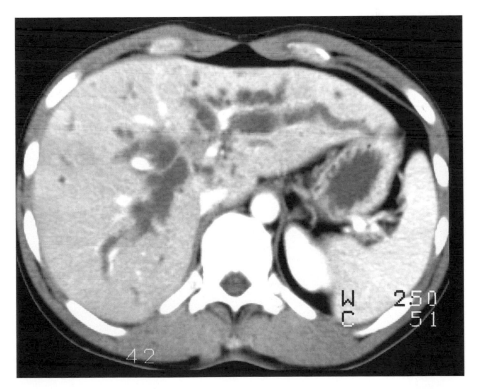

Klatskin's tumor with marked dilatation of intrahepatic bile ducts. Hypodense demarcation of the tumor at the junction of the intrahepatic ducts.

Liver (lesion characterization)

Region	liver lesion
Scout view	256 mm, 120 kV, 50–100 mA, pa
Unenhanced	120 kV, 100 mA, inspiration
	8 mm slice thickness / 8 mm table feed top to bottom
Contrast media	i.v.: 120 ml non-ionic CM, iodine content: 300–320 mg/ml no oral contrast material
Injection rate	4 ml/sec
Scan delay time	15 sec after start of bolus (arterial phase)
CT technique	120 kV, 100–200 mA, 512 matrix, inspiration, localize largest extension of lesion, followed by serial dynamic scanning
	dynamic: 10 mm slice thickness / 0 mm table feed 8 acquisitions every 3 sec, followed by 5 acquisitions every 10 sec, and 1 acquisition each after 2, 3, 4, and 5 min
	instruct patient to breathe after the initial 8 acquisitions, after the following 3, and then before each of the acquisitions at 1 min intervals
Reconstruction	standard algorithm
Photography	12 on 1, patient information, scout view without and with cut lines, soft-tissue window,
Remarks	1. The dynamic CM enhanced study starting in the early arterial phase yields information for lesion characterization (in particular differentiation of FNH, adenoma, HCC, hemangioma). The patient has to be instructed prior to the examination to attain a similar degree of inspiration with each breath-hold for image acquisition at identical locations.
	2. The dynamic study can be evaluated by means of an ROI (region of interest) placed in the lesion and plotting of a time/density curve.
	3. The tube current should not exceed 200 mA per scan to minimize radiation exposure.
	4. Giant lesions may require delayed scanning after 10 min.

Brief protocol
unenhanced **CM i.v.** **120 ml** **4 ml/sec** **15 sec** **dynamic series**

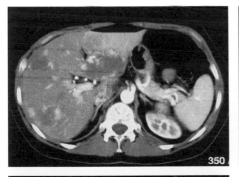

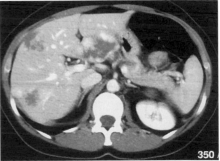

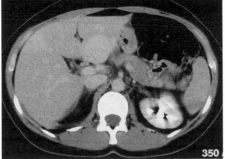

Typical appearance of liver hemangiomas. The serial study shows isolated CM pools in the periphery of the lesions 21 sec after administration of the CM bolus. Increasing enhancement of the center of the lesion 50 sec later ("fill-in phenomenon"). Homogeneous appearance of the liver on the delayed scan.

CT during arterial portography (CTAP)

Region	entire liver
Scout view	256 mm, 120 kV, 50–100 mA, pa
Unenhanced	120 kV, 100–150 mA, inspiration
	10 mm slice thickness / 10 mm table feed top to bottom
Contrast media	i.a.: 60 ml non-ionic CM, iodine content: 300–320 mg/ml mixed 1:1 with 60 ml NaCl solution (total volume 120 ml) injection via intra-arterial catheter with tip in the superior mesenteric artery or splenic artery
Injection rate	2 ml/sec
Scan delay time	15 sec after start of bolus
CT technique	120 kV, 200–300 mA, 512 matrix, inspiration
	10 mm slice thickness / 10 mm table feed top to bottom, entire liver
Reconstruction	standard algorithm
Photography	12 on 1, patient information, scout view without and with cut lines, unenhanced and CM enhanced series at soft-tissue window, basal lung segments at lung window (with edge enhancement if required)
Remarks	CTAP is at present the most sensitive modality for pre-operative detection of liver lesions, but it is not suitable for lesion characterization (see liver protocol for lesion characterization, page 130).

Brief protocol

**unenhanced
CM i.a.
60/60 ml
(CM/NaCl)
2 ml/sec
15 sec
10/10
top to bottom**

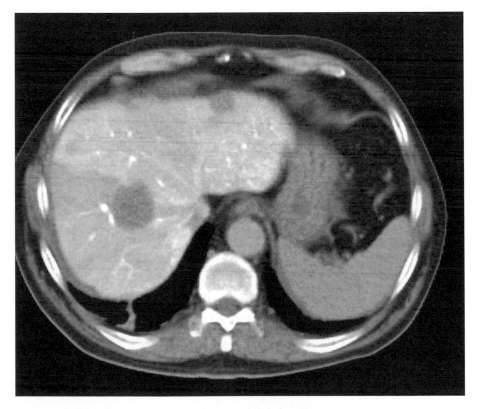

Pre-operative CT for the exclusion of liver metastases from colon carcinoma. Demonstration of two roundish, hypodense lesions in the 2nd and 8th liver segment. Wedge-shaped area of reduced perfusion centrifugal to the lesion in the 8th segment due to vascular compression by the tumor.

Pancreas (pancreatitis, follow-up)

Region	above diaphragm to below uncinate process
Scout view	256 mm, 120 kV, 50–100 mA, pa
Unenhanced	120 kV, 100 mA, inspiration
	8 mm slice thickness / 8 mm table feed top to bottom
Contrast media	i.v.: 100 ml non-ionic CM, iodine content: 300–320 mg/ml oral: 500 ml over 15 min (only if clinically justifiable), the last cup immediately before scanning
Injection rate	2.5 ml/sec
Scan delay time	30 sec after start of bolus
CT technique	120 kV, 200–300 mA, 512 matrix, inspiration
	5 mm slice thickness / 5 mm table feed top to bottom
Reconstruction	standard algorithm
Photography	12 on 1, patient information, scout view without and with cut lines, unenhanced and CM enhanced series at soft-tissue window, basal lung segments at lung window
Remarks	1. Normal tap water or carbonated mineral water can be used as an alternative to positive (radiodense) oral contrast material. This will make the duodenal wall appear bright (CM enhancement) against the lumen. Administer oral CM only if clinically justifiable. 2. Instruct the patient to breathe deeply before scanning. 3. Enhancement as an expression of normal parenchymal perfusion can be quantified by comparing the pre- and post-contrast CT values in an ROI (region of interest) (typical values: post-contrast increase > 30 HU). 4. For oral CM administration, see "General remarks", page IX.

Brief protocol
unenhanced
CM oral, i.v.
100 ml
2.5 ml/sec
30 sec
5/5
top to bottom

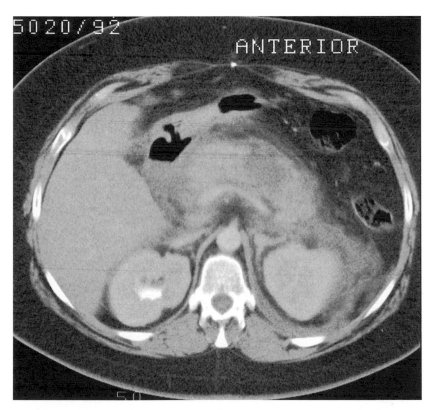

Necrosis of the pancreatic body in a patient with necrotizing pancreatitis. The necrotic tissue is clearly demarcated against the enhanced vital tissue. Extensive peripancreatic exudates extending into the renal fascia on the left.

Pancreas (tumor search, tumor staging)

Region	above diaphragm to below uncinate process
Scout view	256 mm, 120 kV, 50–100 mA, pa
Unenhanced	120 kV, 100 mA, inspiration
	8 mm slice thickness / 8 mm table feed top to bottom
Contrast media	i.v.: 140 ml non-ionic CM, iodine content: 300–320 mg/ml oral: 500 ml over 15 min, the last cup immediately before scanning
Injection rate	4 ml/sec
Scan delay time	30 sec after start of bolus
CT technique	120 kV, 200–300 mA, 512 matrix, inspiration
	5 mm slice thickness / 5 mm table feed top to bottom
Reconstruction	standard algorithm
Photography	12 on 1, patient information, scout view without and with cut lines, unenhanced and CM enhanced series at soft-tissue window, basal lung segments at lung window
Remarks	1. Normal tap water or carbonated mineral water can be used as an alternative to positive (radiodense) oral contrast material. This will make the duodenal wall appear bright (CM enhancement) against the lumen. 2. Instruct the patient to breathe deeply before scanning. 3. In selected cases, it might be advantageous to inject 10–20 mg Glucagon® intravenously for optimal duodenal distension. 4. For oral CM administration, see "General remarks", page IX.

Brief protocol
unenhanced
CM oral, i.v.
140 ml
4 ml/sec
30 sec
5/5
top to bottom

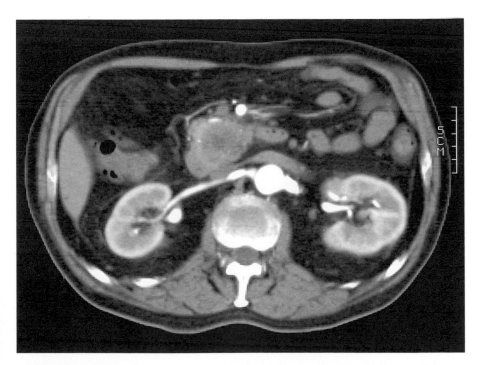

Sonographically suspected malignancy of the uncinate process. With still pronounced arterial opacification and early parenchymal enhancement, the hypodense tumor is seen in the uncinate process. Good demarcation against the superior mesenteric artery; superior mesenteric vein not yet opacified.

Kidneys

Region	kidneys
Scout view	256 mm, 120 kV, 50–100 mA, pa
Unenhanced	120 kV, 100 mA, inspiration
	8 mm slice thickness / 8 mm table feed top to bottom
Contrast media	i.v.: 80 ml non-ionic CM, iodine content: 300–320 mg/ml oral: 1000 ml over 60 min
Injection rate	2 ml/sec
Scan delay time	30 sec after start of bolus
CT technique	120 kV, 100–300 mA, 512 matrix, inspiration
	5 mm slice thickness / 5 mm table feed top to bottom
Reconstruction	standard algorithm
Photography	12 on 1, patient information, scout view without and with cut lines, unenhanced and CM enhanced series at soft-tissue window
Remarks	1. For assessment of suspected thrombosis of the renal vein or inferior vena cava in patients with known malignancy, the scan delay should be 60 sec and the scanning area should extend from the renal vein to the right atrium. 3. Sagittal 2D reconstruction is recommended for assessment of tumor extension. 4. In case of a pathologic finding in the renal pelvis/ureter, delayed scanning with 100–150 mA after 5 min may be necessary. Alternatively, 20 ml contrast material for opacification of the renal pelvis/ureter may be administered about 5 min before scanning.

Brief protocol
unenhanced
CM oral, i.v.
80 ml
2 ml/sec
30 sec
8/8, 5/5
top to bottom

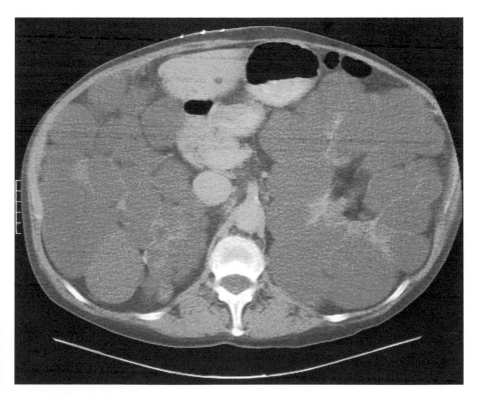

Polycystic renal degeneration (requiring dialysis). Visualization of minimal residual parenchyma after intravenous administration of contrast material.

Adrenal glands

Region	adrenals
Scout view	256 mm, 120 kV, 50–100 mA, pa
Unenhanced	120 kV, 75–150, inspiration
	5 mm slice thickness / 5 mm table feed top to bottom
Contrast media	i.v.: 120 ml non-ionic CM, iodine content: 300–320 mg/ml
Injection rate	2 ml/sec
Scan delay time	40 sec after start of bolus
CT technique	120 kV, 75–200 mA, inspiration
	5 mm slice thickness / 5 mm table feed top to bottom
Reconstruction	standard algorithm magnified reconstruction of scans containing adrenals (smaller FOV)
Photography	12 on 1, patient information, scout view without and with cut lines, unenhanced and CM enhanced series (with magnification if required) at soft-tissue window

Only for adrenal tumors (diameter > 2.5 cm)

Remarks

1. The risk of inducing a hypertensive crisis in patients with pheochromocytoma by intravenous administration of contrast material is discussed controversially in the literature. However, we recommend that phentolamine for intravenous injection (Regitin®) should be readily available for emergencies.
2. In patients with clinically suspected pheochromocytoma and no adrenal abnormalities, scanning should be extended to the area of the aortic bifurcation and, if necessary, to the urinary bladder after CM administration to exclude extra-adrenal localization (Zuckerkandl's organ).
3. The tube current should not exceed 75 mA in slender patients.

Brief protocol
unenhanced
CM i.v.
if required
120 ml
2 ml/sec
40 sec
5/5
top to bottom

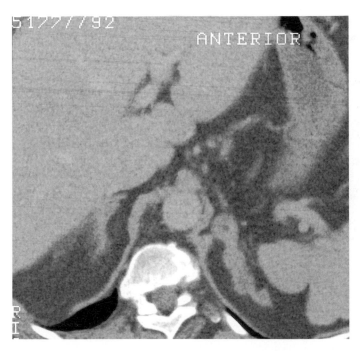

Nodular distension of the left adrenal in a patient with adrenogenital syndrome.

Paranasal sinuses

Region	posterior wall of sphenoidal sinuses to anterior wall of frontal sinuses
Scout view	256 mm, 120 kV, 50 mA, lateral
Contrast media	–
Injection rate	–
Scan delay time	–
CT technique	120 kV, 50–150 mA, 512 matrix
	patient in prone position with reclined head, gantry inclination perpendicular to orbital floor (coronal section)
	5 mm slice thickness / 5 mm table feed posterior to anterior
Reconstruction	lung/bone algorithm
Photography	12 on 1, patient information, scout view without and with cut lines, soft-tissue window, lung window
Remarks	1. Since the lenses are in the scanning area, strict indication and minimal tube current (≤ 50 mA) are mandatory. 2. For pre-operative planning in the area of the anterior ethmoidal cells (orifices!), a slice thickness of 2 mm and an increment of 3 mm may be used. 3. For tumor staging, an axial examination of the frontal skull and neck is recommended after 120 ml of i.v. CM, injection rate 2 ml/sec, 60 sec scan delay, 5/5, as well as coronal reconstruction in the area of the paranasal sinuses.

Brief protocol

**unenhanced
5/5
coronal
low-dose
technique**

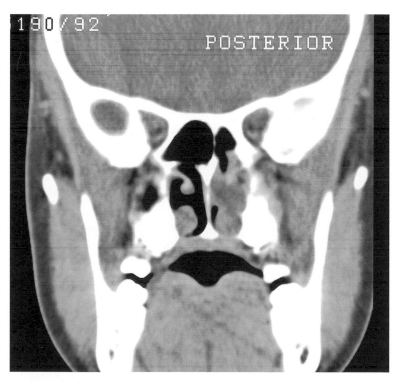

190/92

POSTERIOR

Study of the paranasal sinuses, coronal section: mucosal swelling of the posterior parts of the nasal conchae on the right.

Dental CT (with multiplanar reconstruction)

Region	entire maxilla or mandible, depending on diagnostic problem
Scout view	256 mm, 120 kV, 50 mA, lateral
Contrast media	–
Injection rate	–
Scan delay time	–
CT technique	120 kV, 50 mA, 512 matrix, 2 sec scan time
	patient in supine position with fixed head, gantry inclination parallel to the branch of jaw to be examined, place cellulose or a non-radiodense wedge between teeth
	1.5 mm slice thickness / 1 mm table feed
Reconstruction	lung/bone algorithm
Postprocessing	multiplanar sectioning along row of teeth, coronal (image similar to OPTG) and sagittal (perpendicular to branch of jaw)
Photography	patient information, scout view, 12 on 1 for coronal sections, 36 on 1 for sagittal sections, bone window
Remarks	1. The slice thickness should not be greater than 2 mm since partial volume effects may reduce the delineation of the mandibular canal and other structures.
	2. The energy per section should not exceed 100 mA.
	3. Securely fix the patient's head.

Brief protocol

unenhanced
1.5/1
axial, 50 mA
multiplanar
reconstruction
coronal/sagittal

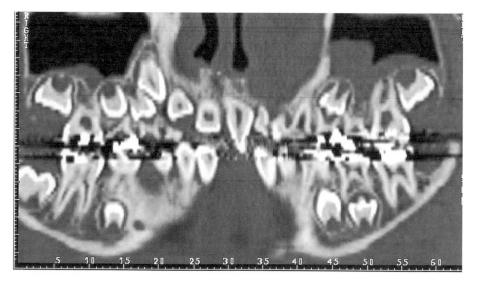

Unclear sinusitis of possible odontogenous origin. In axial orientation, artifacts produced by amalgam fillings are in the horizontal plane.

Thoracic aortic aneurysm (TAA)

Region	above clavicles to below diaphragm
Scout view	512 mm, 120 kV, 50–100 mA, pa
Contrast media	i.v.: 140 ml non-ionic CM, iodine content: 300–320 mg/ml
Injection rate	1.5 ml/sec
Scan delay time	15 sec after start of bolus
CT technique	120 kV, 150–200 mA, 512 matrix, inspiration
	10 mm slice thickness / 10 mm table feed top to bottom
Reconstruction	standard algorithm
Postprocessing	multiplanar coronal and sagittal sectioning
Photography	12 on 1, patient information, scout view without and with cut lines, axial sections at soft-tissue window, reconstructions in pertinent projections.
Remarks	Secondary reconstructions for 3D display of vessel configuration may convey the findings best.

Brief protocol
CM i.v. 140 ml 1.5 ml/sec 15 sec 10/10 top to bottom

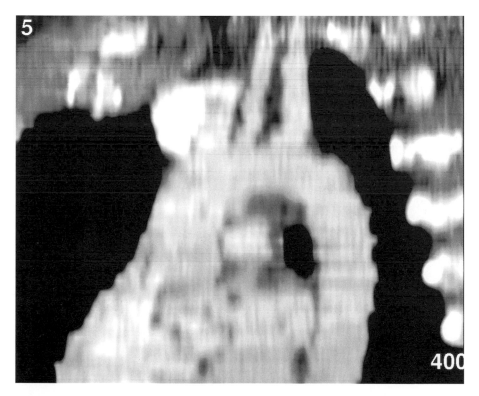

Suspicion of thoracic aortic aneurysm in a patient with acute symptoms of transverse spinal cord lesion. Multiplanar parasagittal reconstruction without signs of aneurysm. The cogwheel-like appearance of the aorta is caused by pulsation artifacts.

Abdominal aortic aneurysm (AAA)

Region	above diaphragm to level of hip joints
Scout view	512 mm, 120 kV, 50–100 mA, pa
Contrast media	i.v.: 140 ml non-ionic CM, iodine content: 300–320 mg/ml
Injection rate	1.5 ml/sec
Scan delay time	15 sec after start of bolus
CT technique	120 kV, 150–200 mA, 512 matrix, inspiration
	10 mm slice thickness / 10 mm table feed top to bottom
Reconstruction	standard algorithm
Postprocessing	multiplanar coronal and sagittal sectioning
Photography	12 on 1, patient information, scout view without and with cut lines, axial images at soft-tissue window, reconstructions in pertinent projections
Remarks	1. Secondary reconstructions for 3D display of vessel configuration may convey the findings best. 2. Do not give oral contrast material since overlying bowel loops filled with contrast material will considerably impair the identification of vessels on reconstructed images.

Brief protocol
CM i.v.
140 ml
1.5 ml/sec
15 sec
10/10
top to bottom

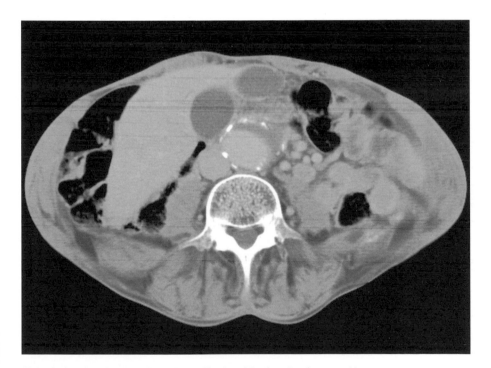

Abdominal aortic aneurysm with weak opacification of the thrombus-free vessel lumen.

Thoracic and abdominal aortic aneurysm

Region	above clavicles to level of hip joints
Scout view	512 mm, 120 kV, 50–100 mA, pa
Contrast media	i.v.: 180 ml non-ionic CM, iodine content: 300–320 mg/ml
Injection rate	1.5 ml/sec
Scan delay time	15 sec after start of bolus
CT technique	120 kV, 150–200 mA, 512 matrix, inspiration 10 mm slice thickness / 10 mm table feed top to bottom
Reconstruction	standard algorithm
Postprocessing	multiplanar coronal and sagittal sectioning
Photography	12 on 1, patient information, scout view without and with cut lines, axial images at soft-tissue window, reconstructions in pertinent projections
Remarks	1. Secondary reconstructions for 3D display of vessel configuration may convey the findings best. 2. Do not give oral contrast material since overlying bowel loops filled with contrast material will considerably impair the identification of vessels on reconstructed images. 3. For assessing the extent of dissection and involvement of aortic branches such as cranial vessels, renal arteries, or mesenteric arteries, these areas should be scanned again at a slice thickness of 5 mm and a table feed of 5 mm. Administration of second contrast bolus: 40 ml, 1 ml/sec, 15 sec scan delay.

Brief protocol
CM i.v.
180 ml
1.5 ml/sec
15 sec
10/10
top to bottom

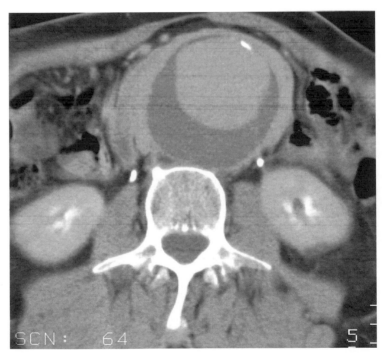

Inflammatory aortic aneurysm with typical wall thickening. Opacified lumen with a semi-circular mural thrombus.

Cardiac CT

Region	aortic arch to apex of heart
Scout view	256 mm, 120 kV, 50–100 mA, lateral
Contrast media	i.v.: 100 ml non-ionic CM, iodine content: 300–320 mg/ml
Injection rate	1.5 ml/sec
Scan delay time	15 sec after start of bolus
CT technique	120 kV, 150–200 mA, 512 matrix, inspiration maximal gantry inclination along the long heart axis 10 mm slice thickness / 10 mm table feed bottom to top
Reconstruction	standard algorithm
Postprocessing	multiplanar sectioning every 3 mm along the long heart axis, corresponding to a coronal heart section
Photography	12 on 1, patient information, scout view without and with cut lines, original images and reconstructions at soft-tissue window, original images at lung window (with edge enhancement if required)
Remarks	1. To facilitate evaluation, axial sections can be calculated from the original data by multiplanar reconstruction. 2. Increase scan delay to 25 sec in patients with known heart failure.

Brief protocol

CM i.v.
100 ml
1.5 ml/sec
15 sec
10/10
bottom to top

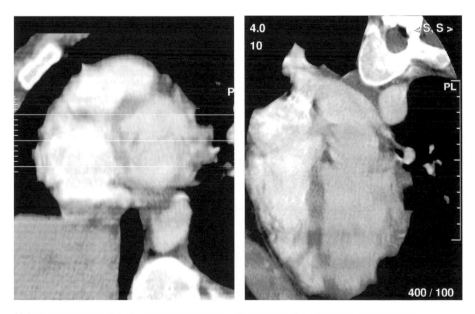

Multiplanar reconstruction along the long heart axis. No demonstration of an intracardiac thrombus.

Gadolinium-DTPA: Neck

Contrast media	i.v.: 60 ml gadolinium-DTPA
Injection rate	2 ml/sec
Scan delay time	25 sec after start of bolus
CT technique	120 kV, 75–150 mA, inspiration incline gantry parallel to intervertebral disc C4–C5 spiral: 5 mm slice thickness / 5 mm table feed (pitch 1:1) top to bottom
Reconstruction	5 mm interval, soft-tissue algorithm
Photography	refer to long-spiral CT protocol for the neck, page 12

Gadolinium-DTPA: Chest

Contrast media	i.v.: 60 ml gadolinium-DTPA
Injection rate	2 ml/sec
Scan delay time	20 sec after start of bolus
CT technique	120 kV, 75–200 mA, inspiration spiral: 10 mm slice thickness / 10 mm table feed (pitch 1:1) bottom to top, sinus to above clavicles
Reconstruction	4 mm interval, lung/bone algorithm
Photography	refer to long-spiral CT protocol for the chest, page 14

Brief protocol
Neck
CM i.v. 60 ml Gd-DTPA 2 ml/sec 25 sec 5/5/5 top to bottom

Brief protocol
Chest
CM i.v. 60 ml Gd-DTPA 2 ml/sec 20 sec 10/10/4 bottom to top

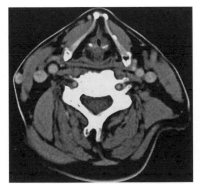 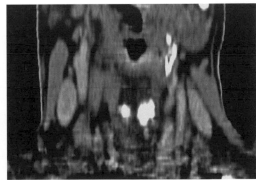

69-year-old male with thyroid cancer. Gadolinium-DTPA was used since radio-iodine therapy was to be carried out. Note the contrast enhanced vasculature that facilitates lymph node detection.

References

1. Brink JA, Heiken JP, Balfe DM, et al.: Spiral CT: decreased spatial resolution in vivo due to broadening of section sensitivity profile. Radiology, 185: 469-474, 1992
2. Brink JA, Lim JT, Wang G, Heiken JP, Deyoe LA, Vannier MW: Technical optimization of spiral CT for depiction of renal artery stenosis: in vitro analysis. Radiology, 194: 157-163, 1995
3. Chambers TP, Baron RL, Lush RM: Hepatic CT enhancement. Part I. Alterations in the volume of contrast material within the same patients. Radiology, 193: 513-517, 1994
4. Chambers TP, Baron RL, Lush RM: Hepatic CT enhancement. Part II. Alterations in contrast material volume and rate of injection within the same patients. Radiology, 193: 518-522, 1994
5. Costello P, Ecker CP, Tello R, Hartnell GG: Assessment of the thoracic aorta by spiral CT. AJR, 158: 1127-1130, 1992
6. Foley WD: Dynamic hepatic CT. Radiology, 170: 617-622, 1989
7. Freeny PC, Nghiem HV, Winter TC: Helical CT during arterial portography: optimization of contrast enhancement and scanning parameters. Radiology, 194: 83-90, 1995
8. Graeter T, Schaefer C, Prokop M, Laas J: Three-dimensional vascular imaging – an additional diagnostic tool. Thorac Cardiovasc Surg, 41: 183-185, 1993
9. Heiken JP, Brink JA, McClennan BL, et al.: Dynamic contrast-enhanced CT of the liver: comparison of contrast medium injection rates and uniphasic and biphasic injection protocols. Radiology, 187: 327-331, 1993
10. Heller CM, Knapp J, Halliday J, O´Connell D, Heller RF: Failure to demonstrate contrast nephrotoxicity. Med J Aust, 155: 329-332, 1991
11. Kalender WA, Polacin A, Suss C: A comparison of conventional and spiral CT: an experimental study on the detection of spherical lesions. JCMT, 18: 167-176, 1994
12. Kalender WA, Polacin A: Physical performance characteristics of spiral CT scanning. Med Phys, 18: 910-915, 1991
13. Kalender WA, Seissler W, Klotz E, et al.: Spiral volumetric CT with single-breath-hold technique, continuous transport, and continuous scanner rotation. Radiology, 176: 181-183, 1990
14. Little AF, Baron RL, Peterson MS, Confer SR, Dodd GD 3rd, Chambers TP, Federle MP, Oliver JH, Orons PD, Sammon JK, et al.: Optimizing CT portography: a prospective comparison of injection into the splenic versus superior mesenteric artery. Radiology, 193: 651-655, 1994
15. Miles KA, McPherson SJ, Hayball MP: Transient splenic inhomogeneity with contrast-enhanced CT: mechanism and effect of liver disease. Radiology, 194: 91-95, 1995
16. Ney DR, Fishman EK, Kawashima A, Robertson DD Jr, Scott WW: Comparison of helical and serial CT with regard to three-dimensional imaging of musculoskeletal anatomy. Radiology, 185: 865-869, 1992
17. Patten RM, Byun JY, Freeny PC: CT of hypervascular hepatic tumors: are unenhanced scans necessary for diagnosis? AJR, 161: 979-984, 1993
18. Polacin A, Kalender WA, Marchal G: Evaluation of section sensitivity profiles and image noise in spiral CT. Radiology, 185: 29-35, 1992
19. Powe NR, Moore RD, Steinberg EP: Adverse reactions to contrast media: factors that determine the cost of treatment. AJR, 161: 1089-1095, 1993
20. Quint LE, Whyte RI, Kazerooni EA, et al.: Stenosis of the central airways: evaluation by using helical CT with multiplanar reconstructions. Radiology, 194: 871-877, 1995
21. Remy J, Remy-Jardin M, Giraud F, Wattinne L: Angioarchitecture of pulmonary arteriovenous malformations: clinical utility of three-dimensional helical CT. Radiology, 191: 657-664, 1994

22. Rubin GD, Dake MD, Napel SA, et al.: Spiral CT of renal artery stenosis: comparison of three-dimensional rendering techniques. Radiology, 190: 181-189, 1994

23. Rubin GD, Dake MD, Napel SA, McDonnell CH, Jeffrey RB Jr: Three-dimensional spiral CT angiography of the abdomen: initial clinical experience. Radiology, 186: 147-152, 1993

24. Schlueter FJ, Wang G, Hsieh PS, Brink JA, Balfe DM, Vannier MW: Longitudinal image deblurring in spiral CT. Radiology, 193: 413-418, 1994

25. Semba CP, Rubin GD, Dake MD: Three-dimensional spiral CT angiography of the abdomen. Semin Ultrasound CT MR, 15: 133-138, 1994

26. Small WC, Nelson RC, Bernardino ME, Brummer LT: Contrast-enhanced spiral CT of the liver: effect of different amounts and injection rates of contrast material on early contrast enhancement. AJR, 163: 87-92, 1994

27. Soyer P, Bluemke DA, Fishman EK: CT during arterial portography for the preoperative evaluation of hepatic tumors: how, when, and why? AJR, 163: 1325-1331, 1994

28. Soyer P, Lacheheb D, Belkacem A, Levesque M: Involvement of superior mesenteric vessels and portal vein in pancreatic adenocarcinoma: detection with CT during arterial portography. Abdom Imaging, 19: 413-416, 1994

29. Urban BA, Fishman EK, Kuhlman JE, Kawashima A, Hennessey JG, Siegelman SS: Detection of focal hepatic lesions with spiral CT: comparison of 4- and 8-mm interscan spacing. AJR, 160: 783-785, 1993

30. Zeman RK, Davros WJ, Berman P, Weltman DI, Silverman PM, Cooper C, Evans SR, Buras BR, Stahl TJ, Nauta RJ, et al.: Three-dimensional models of the abdominal vasculature based on helical CT: usefulness in patients with pancreatic neoplasms. AJR, 162: 1425-1429, 1994

31. Zeman RK, Fox SH, Silverman PM, et al.: Helical (spiral) CT of the abdomen. AJR, 160: 719-725, 1993